# Medical Terms for Nurses

## A QUICK REFERENCE GUIDE

Janet Duffey
RN, MS, APRN, BC

Vice President and Publisher: Maureen McMahon
Editorial Director: Jennifer Farthing
Contributing Editor: Sandy Gade
Production Editor: Karina Cueto
Production Designer: KeithleyAssociates, Inc.
Cover Designer: Carly Schnur

Published by Kaplan Publishing,
a division of Kaplan, Inc.
1 Liberty Plaza, 24th Floor
New York, NY 10006

Printed in the United States of America

July 2007
10   9   8   7   6   5   4   3   2

ISBN-13: 978-1-4195-9954-5

Kaplan Publishing books are available at special quantity discounts to use for sales promotions, employee premiums, or educational purposes. Please email our Special Sales Department to order or for more information at kaplanpublishing@kaplan.com, or write to Kaplan Publishing, 1 Liberty Plaza, 24th Floor, NY, NY 10006.

# Contents

**Introduction**　　v
How to Use This Book　　v
How Medical Words Are Formed　　vii

**1　Glossary**　　1
Alphabetical Listing of Terms　　1

**2　Resource Lists**　　261
Resource Category 1: Anatomy/Physiology　　261
*Figure 1:* Arterial Supply to the Heart
*Figure 2:* Cardiac Conduction System
*Figure 3:* Cardiovascular System, Heart
*Figure 4:* Cardiovascular System, Major Veins
*Figure 5:* Cardiovascular System, Pulse Points
*Figure 6:* Digestive System
*Figure 7:* Endocrine System
*Figure 8:* Excretory System
*Figure 9:* Human Fetus
*Figure 10:* Lymph Node
*Figure 11:* Lymphatic System
*Figure 12:* Muscles, Anterior
*Figure 13:* Muscles, Posterior
*Figure 14:* Nervous System, Brain
*Figure 15:* Nervous System, Cross-Section of Spinal Cord
　　　　and the Components of a Spinal Nerve
*Figure 16:* Nervous System, Neuron
*Figure 17:* Nervous System, Synapse

*Figure 18:* Reproductive System, Female
*Figure 19:* Reproductive System, Male
*Figure 20:* Respiratory System
*Figure 21:* Skeletal System, Bones
*Figure 22:* Skeletal System, Fractures
*Figure 23:* Skeletal System, Intervertebral Foramen
*Figure 24:* Skin
*Figure 25:* Special Sense Organs, Ear
*Figure 26:* Special Sense Organs, Eye

## Resource Category 2: Diseases, Disorders, and Procedures **287**

General Pathology
  Neurological Disorders
  Cancer
  COPD
  Respiratory Diseases
  Diabetes
  Heart Disease
  Parkinson's Disease
  Sexually Transmitted Diseases
  Stroke
Procedures
  Diagnostic
  Surgical

## Resource Category 3: Word Roots, Prefixes, and Suffixes **293**

Word Roots
Prefixes
Suffixes

## 3 Medical Abbreviations **295**
Common Medical Abbreviations **295**

# Introduction

Medical terms are the common language of many health disciplines, including medicine, nursing, physical therapy, social work, and other ancillary health care disciplines. Regardless of the discipline, it is imperative that health professionals use medical terms in a manner that reflects knowledge and efficiency. This book was created for use by teachers, students, and experienced clinicians alike to enhance and to increase their medical term vocabulary.

It is important to note that considerable variation exists in how nurses learn medical terminology in their academic course work. Some schools require a separate medical terminology class, while others use an integrated approach throughout their curriculum. Notwithstanding the debate on how to best prepare nurses for the challenges of clinical practice, the task of mastering ever-evolving medical innovation and associated language is a challenge for all. This resource will attempt to fill the void between initial educational preparation and the realities of constant change and innovation in clinical practice.

Included in the introduction of this book is an explanation of how medical terms are formed. This foundation is the basis for understanding the approximately 3,400 medical terms contained herein, and will provide you with an effective method of increasing your professional vocabulary throughout your career. While it may be tempting to jump to the alphabetized list for a definition, this section also covers the basic elements of medical terms: prefixes, roots, and suffixes.

The 3,400 terms found in Section 1 have been selected for their accuracy and relevance to multiple patients and practice settings; no single practice area or setting has been deliberately excluded. The terms, including prefixes, suffixes, and roots, are listed alphabetically for convenience. Each term is followed by a phonetic pronunciation and brief definition, but plural forms and synonyms are included only when appropriate. Please note that the definitions provided assume some prior knowledge of anatomy, physiology, and pathological or disease states. It is a supplement to knowledge, but not a full-length pathophysiology text.

In the second section of this book, selected terms are categorized in resource lists based on anatomy, pathologies or diseases, and procedures. Diagrams have also been included to clarify structures related to some anatomical terms. The final resource list is a collection of the most common prefixes, word roots, and suffixes. This may well offer the greatest utility in deciphering the numerous permutations of medical conditions, diagnostics, and interventions in the practice of nursing and related disciplines.

Finally, in Section 3 you will find a comprehensive list of common medical abbreviations. Not all have been covered within the 3,400 terms, so you should use this as a supplemental resource.

## ➤ HOW MEDICAL WORDS ARE FORMED

Most medical words are comprised of four basic elements:

- word roots
- combining forms
- prefixes
- suffixes

While not all words are comprised of all four parts, most have at least two. By analyzing and determining the individual meanings of these parts, the total meaning can be derived even when you are not familiar with the exact word. This approach removes the need for endless memorization of terms in relative isolation one from another.

Each of these four elements is discussed in greater detail here.

## Word Roots

A word root is similar to a subject of a sentence. Often derived from Latin or Greek, it defines the main topic or feature of the word. Typically, the root is in the middle, preceded by a prefix and followed by a variation called a combining form and a suffix—more on these later. A root is essential to the subject of the word. Finding the root is the first clue in deciphering multipart medical terms.

Some roots stand alone. For example, *bruit*, *prostate*, *fever*, *alcohol*, and *thyroid* can be used alone, but are more specific when combined with prefixes or suffixes.

### Example:

*Tendon* is the root in the term *tendonitis*. By combining the root with the suffix *-itis*, we add the meaning of "inflammation of the tendon." Therefore, the translation of the term *tendonitis* is reliant on the root term being modified or described by the suffix.

## Prefixes

Prefixes are highly descriptive word parts at the beginning of the term that lend a specific context to the term. A small selection of commonly used prefixes include: *pre-* (before), *post-* (after), *ab-* (move away from center), *ad-* (move toward center), and *pseudo-* (false or similar to).

Common classifications of prefixes include:

- number (e.g., *bi-* meaning two, *quad-* meaning four)

- size (e.g., *mega-* meaning large, *micro-* meaning small)

- directional (e.g., *para-* meaning beside, *ab-* meaning toward the midline)

- organ (e.g., *encephal-* meaning brain, *hepat-* meaning liver)

- quality (e.g., *dys-* meaning painful, difficult, or bad; *neo-* meaning new)

### Example:

*Pseud-* is the prefix in the term *pseudodementia*. By combining *pseud-* with the root *dementia* and using the combining form "o," we create the meaning of "false decreased cognitive function."

## Combining Forms

Joining of prefixes, root terms, and suffixes is accomplished by using a combining vowel; usually the letter "o" to join the two word parts. Combining forms do not have a specific meaning and do not stand alone, but serve to link the two or more word elements into one word.

### Example:

*Endocrine* means "organs secreting directly into bloodstream," and *-logy* means "the study of." The sum meaning of the root and suffix is "the study of organs that secrete directly into the bloodstream." Replacing the "e" at the end of *endocrine* with the linking combining form "o" facilitates joining the two terms into one word with a highly descriptive meaning.

## Suffixes

Located at the end of a word, suffixes modify the meaning of the word root. Within medical terms, a suffix often describes a disease, condition, structure, procedure, or treatment. Additionally, suffixes can indicate parts of speech such as nouns, adjectives, or diminutive expression.

- A noun suffix describes the condition and may be singular or plural. Examples of noun suffixes describing a condition are: *-esis*, *-ia*, and *-ism*. Noun suffixes are also used to name specific areas of clinical specialty. Examples include: *-iatry* (study or practice of a certain area) and *-ist* (specialist in a particular area).

- In their adjective form, suffixes give great meaning to the root term. Suffixes that mean "related or pertaining to" include: *-ac*, *-al*, *-ar*, *-ary*, *-eal*, *-ic*, *-ile*, *-ior*, *-ous*, and *-tic*. There is one combination suffix: *-ical*, which is a combination of *-ic* and *-al*.

- Diminutive suffixes indicate the small size or scale of the term. Examples of diminutive suffixes are: *-y*, *-icle*, *-ole*, *-ule*.

## Forming Medical Terms

Considerable variation exists in the ability to explain medical phenomena using prefixes, roots, and suffixes. The simplest is a stand-alone root, for example, *phobia*. Many terms include at least one prefix, root, and suffix; for example: *hyper / tens / ive*.

The use of two or more prefixes adds both specificity and complexity to the term. For example: *chol / angio / pancreato / graphy* means "the study of pancreas and bile ducts using x-rays." Terms with this level of complexity are often used to describe a multisystem condition's symptoms, or diagnostic and operative interventions.

## Rules for Combining Forms

1. Word roots link a suffix beginning with a vowel.

   *Example:* [append- + -ectomy] becomes *appendectomy*

2. Combining forms where the suffix begins with a consonant is the root word + "o."

   *Example:* [gynec + o] + *mastia* = *gynecomastia* (gynec/o becomes the combining form)

3. Compound words are formed by linking two root words with "o" in the middle, even when the second root begins with a vowel.

   *Example:* [oste- + o] + *arthritis* = *osteoarthritis*

4. No vowel is added when the suffix begins with a vowel.

   *Example:* *gastro-* + *-itis* = *gastritis*

5. Plural forms of words are dictated by the last letter(s) of the singular form. This rule is demonstrated in the table below.

## From Singular to Plural Forms

Changing a singular form to the plural form entails modification of the suffix. The following table summarizes the rules for conversion of common singular to plural suffixes. Example terms demonstrating the change from singular to plural are provided.

| Singular Suffix | Plural Suffix | Rule for Conversion | Singular to Plural Examples |
|---|---|---|---|
| *-a* | *-ae* | Keep the "a," add "e" | scapula to scapulae |
| *-ax* | *-aces* | Remove "x," add "ces" | pneumothorax to pneumothoraces |
| *-en* | *-ina* | Remove "en," add "ina" | foramen to foramina |
| *-ex* | *-ices* | Remove "ex," add "ices" | apex to apices |
| *-is* | *-es* | Remove "is," add "es" | diagnosis to diagnoses |

| Singular Suffix | Plural Suffix | Rule for Conversion | Singular to Plural Examples |
|---|---|---|---|
| *-ix* | *-ices* | Remove "ix," add "ices" | calix to calices |
| *-ma* | *-mata* *-mas* | Keep "ma," add "ta" OR Add "s" to the end | chondroma to chondromata fibromyoma to fibromyomas |
| *-nx* | *-nges* | Remove "x," add "ges" | phalanx to phalanges |
| *-on* | *-a* | Remove "on," add "a" | ganglion to ganglia |
| *-um* | *-a* | Remove "um," add "a" | bacterium to bacteria |
| *-us* | *-i* | Remove "us," add "i" | sulcus to sulci |
| *-y* | *-ies* | Remove "y," add "ies" | biopsy to biopsies |

## ABCs of Quick Term Definitions

1. **A**nalyze the word parts (prefix, root, suffix)

2. **B**ring the word-part definitions into the order of: suffix, prefix, and root or combining form.

3. **C**omplete the conceptual definition by adding words to link the definitions into a descriptive phrase. For example, *gastroenteritis* would be interpreted by word parts as "stomach, small intestine, inflammation." Rearranged into logical order, it becomes: "inflammation of the stomach and small intestine."

## Conclusion

By mastering the basic building blocks and a few rules, effective communication using medical terms can be used to produce quality patient care across many disciplines. When the exact definition isn't known by rote memorization, these analytic skills provide valuable clues to accurate definitions.

# Glossary

1

## ➤ ALPHABETICAL LISTING OF TERMS

**17-ketosteroids test** [17 kee-toh-STEER-oidz test] a 24-hour urine test to detect steroidal metabolites of androgenic and adrenocortical hormones

**3-methoxy-4-hydroxymandelic acid test** [3 meth-OK-see 4 high-DROK-see-man-DEL-ick as-id test] urine test to detect possible muscular dystrophy

## A

**a-** [ah] *prefix;* without

**ab-** [ab] *prefix;* away from

**abdominal** [ab-DOM-ih-nal] pertaining to the abdomen

**abdominal aorta** [ab-DOM-ih-nal aye-OR-tah] major blood vessel supplying blood to the abdominal organs

**abdominal hernia** [ab-DOM-ih-nal HUR-nee-uh] abnormal protrusion of an organ through the abdominal musculature

**abdominopelvic** [ab-DOM-ih-noh-PEL-vik] pertaining to the region of the body including the abdomen, pelvis (including the renal pelvis), and hip bone

**abduction** [ab-DUK-shun] to draw away from

**aberrant conduction** [AB-er-ant kon-DUKT-shun] passage of electrical impulses of the heart through abnormal pathways

**aberratio testis** [ab-er-AYE-shee-oh test-eez] location of a testicle in an abnormal anatomical position

**ablation** [ab-LAY-shun] destruction of tissue or function by surgery, electrocautery, or radio frequency

**-able** [uh-bul] *suffix*; able to be

**ablepharia** [ab-leh-FAY-ree-ah] congenital defect of eyelid formation, eyelid is either absent or reduced in size

**ablepsia** [ah-BLEP-see-ah] inability to see; blindness

**abrasion** [ah-BRAY-zhun] wearing down of a surface, such as skin, by rubbing or scraping

**abruptio placenta** [ah-BRUP-shee-oh pla-SEN-tah] sudden and premature separation of the placenta from the site of uterine attachment due to bleeding between the placenta and uterine wall

**abscess** [AB-sess] a cavity containing pus and surrounded by inflamed tissue

**absence seizure** [AB-senz SEE-zur] brain dysfunction involving a brief loss of consciousness without motor involvement; also called petit-mal seizure

**absorption** [ab-SORP-shun] process by which digested food nutrients move through villi of the small intestine into the blood

**abstinence** [AB-sti-nenz] refraining from certain behaviors, activities, foods, or beverages

**abstract** [AB-strakt] summary statement of research article that identifies the purpose, methodology, findings, and conclusions

**abulia** [ah-BYOO-lee-ah] impaired ability to make decisions, perform voluntary actions, react emotionally or verbally; commonly associated with bilateral frontal lobe disease

**ac-** [ak] *prefix*; pertaining to

**acantha** [ah-KAN-tha] general term for spine, especially the spinous process of a vertebra

**acanthosis** [ak-an-THOH-sis] breakdown or separation of the prickle-cell layer of the epidermis leading to cellular degeneration

**acataphasia** [ah-kat-ah-FAY-zee-ah] an inability to choose words that accurately reflect thoughts and/or to speak correct words due to a cerebral lesion

**accommodation** [ah-com-moh-DAY-shun] adaptation or adjustment to physical or psychological changes; adjustment of the eye to focus on objects at various distances

**acet-** [as-eet] *prefix*; vinegar; acid; sour; sharp

**acetabulum** [as-ee-TAB-yoo-lum] a cup-shaped socket in the hip bone, formed by the ilium, that is occupied by the head of the femur, forming the hip joint

**acetylcholine** [as-ee-til-KOH-leen] chemical involved in nerve impulse transmission

**Achilles reflex** [ah-KIL-eez REE-flecks] contraction of the calf muscle following a sharp blow to the Achilles tendon behind the ankle

**Achilles tendon** [ah-KIL-eez TEN-don] tendon of the lower leg that extends from the gastrocnemius and soleus muscles and attaches to the calcaneus bone of the heel; it is the thickest and strongest tendon of the body

**achillorrhaphy** [ah-kil-OR-ah-fee] surgical repair of the Achilles tendon by suturing

**acidosis** [as-ih-DOH-sis] an abnormal increase in hydrogen ion concentration in the body

**acne vulgaris** [AK-nee vul-GAIR-ris] inflammation of the hair follicle and associated sebaceous glands

**acoustic neuroma** [ah-KOOS-tik nyoo-ROH-mah] benign tumor of the vestibulocochlear nerve resulting in pain, headache, hearing loss, tinnitus, and disturbed balance

**acquired immunodeficiency syndrome (AIDS)** [ah-kwyrd IM-yoo-noh-dee-FISH-en-see SIN-drom] syndrome of immune disruption with opportunistic diseases such as pneumonia, Kaposi's sarcoma, and others due to infection with human immunodeficiency virus by sexual contact and blood-borne exposure

**acromegaly** [ak-roh-MEG-ah-lee] excessive secretion of the growth hormone somatotropin that produces enlargement of head, face, hands, and feet

**acromion** [ah-KROH-mee-on] a long, bladelike spine along the upper half of the scapula bone

**acrotism** [ak-ROH-tizm] having an undetectable pulse

**actin** [AK-tin] a muscle protein that is responsible for muscle contraction

**actinic keratosis** [ak-TIN-ik ker-ah-TOH-sis] localized thickening and scaling of the outer layers of the skin as a result of prolonged exposure to the sun

**actinotherapy** [AK-tin-oh-THER-ah-pee] treatment of skin disorders using rays such as ultraviolet radiation

**action potential** [AK-shun poh-TEN-shul] the change in electrical charge within a nerve or muscle when stimulated

**activated charcoal** [AK-ti-vay-ted CHAR-kol] an agent given by mouth or nasogastric tube to absorb toxic substances in the stomach

**active euthanasia** [AK-tiv yoo-tha-NAY-zee-ah] process of taking deliberate action that will hasten the client's death

**acupressure** [AK-yoo-pres-shur] use of finger pressure applied to specific nerve junctions on the body to promote healing

**-acusis** [ah-koo-sis] *suffix*; related to hearing

**acute** [ah-KYOOT] intense, sharp, severe symptoms followed by a short course of illness

**acute crisis** [ah-KYOOT KRI-sis] severe state of disorganization that occurs when the individual's usual coping mechanisms, physical or emotional, are no longer effective

**acute pain** [ah-KYOOT payn] discomfort identified by sudden onset and relatively short duration, mild to severe intensity, and a steady decrease in intensity over several days or weeks

**acute respiratory distress syndrome** [ah-KYOOT RES-pih-ra-tore-ee dis-TRES SIN-drom] massive damage to alveoli due to injury to lungs from burns, aspiration of vomitus, or infection which renders the lungs incapable of making surfactant required to keep lung tissue open

**ad-** [ad] *prefix*; toward midline or near

**-ad** [ahd] *suffix*; toward or in direction of

**adaptation** [ad-ap-TAY-shun] component of cognitive development that refers to the changes that occur as a result of assimilation and accommodation; ongoing process by which an individual adjusts to stressors in order to achieve homeostasis

**addiction** [ah-DIK-shun] a state of complete physical and psychological dependence on a substance

**Addison's disease** [AD-dih-suns dis-EEZ] chronic adrenocortical insufficiency possibly due to autoimmune disease, adrenal tumors, or tuberculosis

**adductor longus muscle** [a-DUCK-tur LONG-us MUS-sel] muscle of the thigh and one of five medial femoral muscles; it functions to adduct and flex the thigh

**adductor magnus muscle** [a-DUCK-tur MAG-nus MUS-sel] muscle of the medial aspect of the thigh which acts to adduct the thigh; the proximal portion acts to rotate the thigh medially and to flex it on the hip

**-ade** [ayd] *suffix*; action or process

**adenitis** [ad-eh-NY-tis] inflammation of a gland or lymph node

**adenocarcinoma** [AD-eh-ooh-KAR-sih-NOH-mah] cancer tumor, mass gland

**adenohypophysis** [ad-ee-noh-high-POF-ih-sis] anterior pituitary gland, which produces hormones

**adenoids** [AD-en-oydz] lymphatic tissue on the back of the nasopharynx; also called pharyngeal tonsil

**adenosine** [ah-DEN-oh-seen] a highly potent vasodilator used to perform cardiovascular perfusion studies without having the client exercise

**adenosine monophosphate** [ah-DEN-oh-seen mon-oh-FOS-fayt] a hormone secreted by the parafocicular cells of the thyroid gland to regulate the level of blood calcium

**adenosine triphosphate (ATP)** [ah-DEN-oh-seen try-FOS-fate] a molecular substance that supplies the energy for muscle fiber contraction; energy is released when ATP is hydrolyzed to adenosine diphosphate

**adenovirus** [AD-eh-noh-VY-rus] a large group of viruses causing common colds and upper respiratory tract infections

**adherence** [ad-HEER-ents] the degree of compliance or continuance of a therapeutic action; ability of two surfaces to stick together

**adhesion** [ad-HEE-zhun] abnormal fibrous bands of tissue that form after abdominal or other surgeries

**adipose** [AD-ih-poze] fat

**adipsia** [ah-DIP-see-ah] lack of normal thirst

**adjustment disorder** [ad-JUST-ment dis-OR-der] psychiatric illness characterized by gross inability to effectively respond to a major stressful life event

**adnexa** [ad-NEK-sa] connecting parts of a structure; as demonstrated in the uterine adnexa, which includes the uterine tubes, ovaries, and uterine ligaments

**adrenal cortex** [ah-DREE-nal KOHR-tex] outer portion of the adrenal gland

**adrenal glands** [ah-DREE-nal glanz] endocrine gland located on each kidney; comprised of the adrenal cortex, which excretes steroid hormones, and the adrenal medulla, which secretes epinephrine and norepinephrine

**adrenal medulla** [ah-DREE-nal me-DEW-luh] inner portion of the adrenal gland

**adrenal virilism** [ah-DREE-nal VIR-ih-lizm] masculine facial and body features in females due to hypersecretion of androgens

**adrenalectomy** [ah-dree-nal-EK-toh-mee] surgical removal of the adrenal gland

**adrenaline** [ah-DREN-ah-lin] epinephrine; hormone secreted by the adrenal medulla

**adrenocortical steroid hormone** [ah-DREE-noh-KOR-ti-kal STEER-oyd HOR-mohn] hormones, including glucocorticoids, mineralocorticoids, and androgens, that are produced by the adrenal cortex

**adrenocorticotropic hormone (ACTH)** [ah-DREE-noh-kor-tih-koh-TROP-ik HOR-mohn] a hormone secreted by the pituitary gland that stimulates the release of hormones from the renal cortex

**advance directive** [ad-VANCE DYE-rek-tiv] written instruction for health care that is recognized under state law and is used in the provision of such care when the individual is incapacitated

**adventitious breath sounds** [ad-ven-TISH-us breth sownds] abnormal sounds, such as crackles and rhonchi, heard in the lungs during auscultation

**adverse reaction** [ad-VERS re-AK-shun] drug effect contrary to what is therapeutically intended

**aer-** [er] *prefix*; gas or air

**aerobic metabolism** [air-RO-bik me-TAB-oh-lizm] processing of nutrients in the presence of oxygen; a metabolic pathway that uses oxygen to convert glucose into cellular energy

**aerocele** [ER-oh-seel] distention of a bodily cavity with gas

**aerocoly** [er-OK-oh-lee] distention of the colon with gas

**aerocystoscopy** [er-oh-sis-TOS-koh-pee] visual examination of the bladder using a cystoscope while the bladder is distended by air

**aerophagia** [air-oh-FAY-jee-ah] swallowing air during eating or drinking liquids

**affect** [AF-fekt] outward display on the face

**affective disorder** [ah-FEK-tiv dis-OR-der] a psychiatric condition characterized by disturbance of mood; most commonly depression or anxiety

**affective domain** [af-FEK-tiv doe-MAIN] area of learning that involves attitudes, beliefs, and emotions

**afferent** [AF-fer-ent] to transport or carry toward the center; nerves that return impulses to the central nervous system

**afferent lymphatic vessel** [AF-fer-ent lim-FAT-ik VES-el] a small structure that transports lymph from the periphery or distal portions of the body, draining into more central vessels or lymph nodes

**afferent nerve** [AF-fer-ent nerv] any nerve that transmits impulses from receptors in the peripheral nervous system to the central nervous system; opposite of an efferent nerve

**agglutination** [ah-gluh-tih-NAY-shun] the clumping together of cells as a result of interaction with specific antibodies called agglutinins; agglutinins are used in blood tests that determine the blood type—such as A, B, AB, and O—and Rh factor (positive or negative); derived from a Latin word meaning "glue together"

**aggregates** [AG-gre-gates] individuals, families, and other subgroupings of people who are associated because of singular social, personal, or health care needs; a group or population

**agnosia** [ag-NOH-see-ah] loss of the ability to comprehend sensory input despite normal sensory function

**agonist** [AG-on-ist] pharmacological agent that combines with receptors to initiate drug actions

**agoraphobia** [AG-or-ah-FOH-bee-ah] fear of crowds or public places which causes individuals to resist leaving home even for important or urgent medical care

**-agra** [ag-rah] *suffix*; sudden, severe pain

**agranulocytosis** [aye-GRAN-yoo-loh-sigh-TOH-sis] acute, life-threatening immunocompromised state characterized by severe depression or complete absence of disease-fighting white blood cells and by leukopenia, resulting in infections of the skin and mucous membranes

**agraphia** [aye-GRAF-ee-ah] inability to write due to cerebral pathology

**air embolism** [air EM-bo-lizm] entrance of air into a blood vessel, most often a vein, during trauma or medical procedures; if the amount of air is large enough, death can result

**airborne precautions** [air-born pre-KAW-shuns] actions taken to stop transmission of infectious agents by exposure to airborne droplet spray, including air filtration systems and masks

**air-puff tonometry** [air-puff ton-OM-eh-tree] assessment of intraocular pressure using a burst of air rebounding off the cornea without the instrument touching the patient's eye

**-al** [ul] *suffix*; pertaining or related to

**alanine aminotransferase test** [AL-uh-neen ah-mee-noh-TRANS-fer-ace test] blood enzyme test to evaluate tissue damage

**alarm reaction** [ah-LARM ree-AK-shun] initial phase of general adaptation syndrome; bodily response to stress by release of endocrine hormones preparing for fight or flight

**alb-** [alb] *prefix*; white color, or lacking of normal pigments

**Albert's disease** [AL-bertz dis-EEZ] bursitis of the Achilles tendon with or without calcification; due to trauma or poorly fitting shoes

**albinism** [AL-bih-nizm] hereditary absence of melanin pigment in the body

**albino** [al-BI-noh] lacking pigmentation of the skin, eyes, and hair

**albumin** [al-BEW-min] a major protein molecule in the blood produced by the liver

**albuminuria** [al-bew-mi-NEW-ree-ah] abnormal presence of the protein albumin in the urine

**Alcock's canal** [AL-koks kah-NAL] space in the pelvis between the obturator internus muscle and the obturator fascia that the pudendal nerve passes through

**alcoholic cirrhosis** [al-ko-HOL-ik sir-ROH-sis] liver enlargement, fatty deposits, and fibrosis due to chronic ethanol abuse

**aldosterone** [al-DOS-ter-ohn] a mineralocorticoid steroid hormone that stimulates the renal tubule in the kidneys to retain water and sodium

**-algia** [ahl-jee-ah] *suffix*; painful condition

**algophobia** [al-go-FO-bee-ah] morbid or excessive fear and sensitivity to pain

**algor mortis** [AL-gore MOHR-tis] lack of skin elasticity as a result of death

**algorithm** [AL-go-rith-im] a formula or set of rules for diagnosis and treatment of a disease

**alimentary canal** [al-ih-MEN-tar-ee kah-NAL] gastro-intestinal system including all structures from the mouth to the anus

**alimentation** [al-ih-men-TAY-shun] giving of food or nourishment to the body by natural or artificial means such as feeding tubes or intravenous injection

**-alis** [ah-lis] *suffix;* pertaining or related to

**alkaline phosphatase test** [AL-kah-line FAWS-fah-tace] blood test for the enzyme alkaline phosphatase that is found in both liver cells and bone cells; elevated blood levels are suggestive of liver or bone disease

**alkalosis** [al-ka-LOW-sis] an abnormal condition of body fluids, characterized by a tendency toward a blood pH level greater than 7.45; this level is caused by an excess of alkaline bicarbonate or deficiency of acid

**alkalosis, compensated** [al-ka-LOW-sis, KOM-pen-say-ted] metabolic state where the pH of the blood has returned to normal with increased level of bicarbonate in the blood

**alkalosis, hypochloremic** [al-ka-LOW-sis, hy-po-klo-REE-mik] metabolic state of increased pH of the blood due to loss of chloride; associated with aggressive diuresis, severe vomiting, and drainage of gastric acid by nasogastric tube

**alkalosis, hypokalemic** [al-ka-LOW-sis, hy-po-ka-LEE-mik] metabolic state of increased pH of the blood due to excessive loss of potassium; often associated with diuretic therapy

**alkalosis, metabolic** [al-ka-LOW-sis, met-ah-BOL-ik] metabolic state where bicarbonate levels of the blood are increased resulting from loss of acid from the gastrointestinal tract or kidney, diuretic therapy, intake of alkaline foods, or adrenal gland hyperactivity

**alkalosis, respiratory** [al-ka-LOW-sis, RES-pih-ra-tore-ree] metabolic state where pH of the blood is increased due to hyperventilation resulting in decreased carbon dioxide and subsequent reduction of plasma bicarbonate levels

**Allen test** [AL-len test] procedure that measures the collateral circulation to the radial artery

**allergenic extract** [al-er-JEN-ik EKS-trakt] protein substance from various foods, pollens, and other sources for the purpose of skin testing and desensitization

**allergic rhinitis** [ah-LER-jik rye-NIGH-tis] nasal mucous membrane inflammation caused by allergen inhalation; allergies may be seasonal or year-round

**allo-** [al-oh] *prefix*; referring to another

**allodynia** [AL-oh-dye-nee-uh] pain caused by a stimulus that does not normally evoke pain

**allogeneic** [AL-oh-jeh-NEE-ik] bone marrow, stem cells, or other tissue donated by another person

**allograft** [AL-oh-graft] frozen or freeze-dried bone taken from a cadaver

**allopathic** [AL-oh-path-ik] medical treatments recognized by a specific culture as being traditional, conventional, or mainstream; for example, Western medicine

**alopecia** [al-oh-PEE-shee-ah] partial or complete lack of hair; partial lack on scalp and face (areata); complete lack on scalp (totalis); complete lack of any body hair (universalis)

**alpha waves** [AL-fah wayvz] brain waves typical of a person who is awake and at rest

**alternative medicine** [al-TER-nah-tiv MED-ih-sin] treatment approaches that are not accepted by mainstream Western medical practice, such as acupuncture, chiropractics, hypnosis, etc.

**alveolar hypoventilation** [al-VEE-oh-lar hy-po-ven-tih-LAY-shun] inability to fully expand and fill the small hollow cavities of the lungs

**alveoli** [al-VEE-oh-lie] hollow, sphere-shaped cells of the lung that function to exchange oxygen and carbon dioxide

**Alzheimer's disease** [AWL-zye-murz dis-EEZ] a degenerative brain disorder that causes dementia and physical deterioration with typical onset late in life; disrupts brain function by formation of amyloid plaques, neurofibrillary tangles, and cerebral atrophy

**ambi-** [am-bi] *prefix;* both or two ways

**amblyopia** [am-blee-OH-pee-ah] impaired vision that is unrelated to an ocular lesion and cannot be fully corrected with glasses; most likely cause is abnormal vision during developmental years

**amebiasis** [am-eh-BY-ah-sis] infection with *Entamoeba histolytica* that is spread by ingestion of contaminated food

**amenorrhea** [ah-men-oh-REE-ah] absence of menstruation

**amnesia** [am-NEE-zee-ah] partial or total loss of long-term memory due to trauma or disease of hippocampus

**amniocentesis** [AM-nee-oh-sen-TEE-sis] transabdominal needle aspiration of amniotic fluid from the amniotic sac for diagnostic purposes

**amnion** [AM-nee-on] a thin, transparent, internal fetal membrane that contains the amnionic fluid and fetus during pregnancy

**amniorrhexis** [am-nee-or-REK-sis] rupture of the amnion

**amniotome** [AM-nee-oh-tohm] instrument used to puncture the amnionic membrane

**amniotomy** [am-nee-OT-oh-mee] surgical incision of the amnion to induce labor

**amphi-** [am-fee] *prefix;* both sides or double

**amphiarthrosis** [am-fee-ar-THRO-sis] a slightly moveable joint where the surfaces of the opposing bones are connected by cartilage, as seen in the symphysis pubis

**amputation** [am-pyoo-TAY-shun] removal of an extremity due to trauma or circulatory disease; classified as traumatic or surgical depending on the circumstances in which removal occurred

**amputee** [AM-pyoo-tee] an individual who has lost an extremity or phalange

**amygdaloid body** [ah-MIG-dah-loyd boh-DEE] an almond-shaped area of grey, unmyelinated nerve tissue located in each temporal lobe that plays a major role in processing memory and sensing dangerous situations

**amyl-** [am-il] *prefix*; starch

**amylase** [AM-ih-lays] an enzyme that breaks starch down into smaller carbohydrates; found in starch and pancreatic juice

**amyotrophic lateral sclerosis (ALS)** [aye-mee-oh-TROH-fik LAT-er-ahl skle-ROH-sis] an idiopathic degenerative disease of upper and lower motor neurons, causing motor weakness and spastic limbs; commonly known as Lou Gehrig's disease

**an-** [an] *prefix*; without, not

**ana-** [ah-nah] *prefix*; up or apart, excessive

**anabolism** [ah-NAB-oh-lizm] constructive phase of metabolism

**anacusis** [an-ah-KOO-sis] total deafness

**anaerobic metabolism** [an-er-OH-bik me-TAB-oh-lizm] a process of converting glucose into energy in the absence of oxygen

**analgesia** [an-al-JEE-zee-uh] condition of not experiencing any pain sensation

**analyte** [AN-ah-lyte] any substance that is measured, usually applied to a component of blood or other body fluid; substance dissolved in a solution; also called solute

**anamnestic response** [an-am-NES-tik REE-spons] immune reaction due to formation of antibodies to a pathogenic organism

**anaphia** [an-AH-fee-ah] inability to perceive the sensation of touch

**anaphylaxis** [an-uh-fil-AK-sis] extreme, immediate, hypersensitive reaction to an antigen, protein, or drug with systemic effects including bronchospasm, peripheral edema, and laryngeal edema; these effects may be life threatening

**anaplasia** [an-ah-PLAY-ze-ah] a term applied to cancerous cells that revert to a less developed state in arrangement and structure; a loss of differentiation among cells

**anastomosis** [ah-NAS-toh-MO-sis] to connect two vessels, often blood vessels or bowel segments, to allow continuous flow

**anatomical position** [AN-ah-TOM-ih-kal poe-ZIH-shun] body positioned erect, standing, facing forward, arms at sides, palms forward, and toes pointing forward

**anatomy** [ah-NAT-oh-mee] study of structures of the human body

**-ance** [ans] *suffix*; state of

**ancillary** [AN-sih-lair-ee] accessory or secondary

**-ancy** [an-cee] *suffix*; state of

**androgens** [AN-droh-jinz] hormone promoting male secondary sex characteristics

**anemia** [ah-NEE-mee-ah] reduction in the amount of hemoglobin in the blood, thus decreasing the oxygen-carrying capacity of the blood

**anesthesia** [AN-es-THEE-zee-ah] pharmacological agents used to block nerve sensations

**aneurysm** [AN-yoo-riz-um] a localized dilation of the wall of a blood vessel

**ang-** [anj] *prefix*; distress, choke

**angina pectoris** [an-JYE-nah PECK-tor-is] chest pain that radiates to the left shoulder

**angiocatheter** [AN-jee-oh-KATH-eh-ter] a hollow, flexible tube inserted into a blood vessel to withdraw or instill fluids

**angioedema** [AN-jee-oh-eh-DEE-ma] sudden, well-defined, large area of edema often due to an allergy to foods or drugs

**angiogenesis** [an-jee-oh-JEN-eh-sis] formation of new blood vessels

**angiogram** [AN-jee-oh-gram] radiographic visualization after injecting a radiopaque contrast dye into the bloodstream, enabling the vessels to be "mapped," and identifying areas of narrowing or blockage

**angioplasty** [AN-jee-oh-plas-tee] surgical intervention of diseased vessels for recanalization of a blood vessel; balloon dilation, mechanical stripping, injection of fibrinolytics, or placement of a stint

**angiosarcoma** [AN-jee-oh-sar-KOH-ma] malignant tumor of blood vessels

**angiospasm** [AN-jee-oh-spazm] sudden, painful, involuntary contraction of the muscles associated with the blood vessels

**angiostenosis** [an-jee-oh-steh-NOH-sis] narrowed lumen of a blood vessel

**angiotensin I** [an-jee-oh-TEN-sin won] a physically inactive hormone that is a converted into angiotensin II by the lungs

**angiotensin II** [an-jee-oh-TEN-sin too] a hormone that increases blood pressure and stimulates production and secretion of aldosterone

**anhedonia** [AN-hee-DOH-nee-ah] inability to experience pleasure from any activity

**anicteric** [AN-ik-TER-ik] appearance of being without jaundice

**anions** [AN-eye-onz] ions with a negative charge

**anisocoria** [an-EYE-soh-KO-ree-ah] unequal sizes of the pupils, often caused by glaucoma, head trauma, stroke, or a tumor that causes the iris to dilate and constrict

**anisocytosis** [an-EYE-soh-sy-TOH-sis] an increase in variation of the size of cells, frequently used in reference to red blood cells

**ankylosing spondylitis** [ang-kih-LOH-sing SPAWN-dih-LYE-tis] chronic inflammation of the vertebrae that leads to fibrosis, restricted movement of the vertebrae, and stiffening of the spine; treatment includes nonsteroidal anti-inflammatory agents

**annulus fibrosis** [AN-yoo-lus figh-BRO-sus] layer of fibrocartilage surrounding each intervertebral disc

**anorexia** [an-oh-REK-see-ah] loss of appetite

**anorexia nervosa** [an-oh-REK-see-ah nur-VOH-suh] disorder characterized by not eating due to a morbid fear of weight gain, resulting in severe emaciation

**anosmia** [an-OZ-mee-ah] loss of the sense of smell

**ant-** [ant] *prefix*; apart or excessive

**antacids** [ant-AS-idz] agents used to neutralize acids, most commonly in the stomach

**ante-** [an-tee] *prefix*; before

**ante cibum (a.c.)** [AHN-tee cee-BUM] abbreviated a.c. when written in medical instructions or physician orders, this indicates that medication or treatment is administered before meals

**anteflexion** [an-tee-FLECK-shun] bending forward a part of an organ; normal position of the uterus as it bends forward over the bladder

**anterior** [an-TEER-ee-or] front of the body

**anterior chamber of the eye** [an-TEER-ee-or CHAM-ber uv the eye] area immediately behind the cornea and in front of the lens of the eye

**anterior cruciate ligament** [an-TEER-ee-or KROO-shee-ayt LIG-ah-ment] a band of strong fibrous tissue originating on the front of the femur and inserting on the tibia, acting to stabilize the knee; injuries to this area of the knee are common in athletes

**anterior tibial muscle** [an-TEER-ee-or TIB-ee-al MUS-sel] muscle of front surface of the lower leg that flexes and abducts the foot when contracted

**anterior tibial vein** [an-TEER-ee-or TIB-ee-al vayn] blood vessel that returns blood to the femoral vein from the lower leg

**anterograde amnesia** [AN-ter-oh-grayd am-NEE-zee-ah] lack of ability to recall events after a specific event such as a trauma or administration of a medication

**anteroposterior** [AN-ter-oh-pohs-TEER-ee-or] from the front to the back of the body

**anteversion** [an-tee-VER-shun] forward tilting of organ or part of an organ; forward tilting of uterus over the bladder

**anthracosis** [an-thruh-KOH-sis] lung disease caused by inhalation of coal dust; also known as "black lung disease"

**anthropometric measurements** [an-thro-po-MET-trik MEH-zur-mentz] measurement of the size, weight, and proportions of the body

**anti-** [an-tee] *prefix*; opposed or against

**antianaphylaxis** [an-tee-an-ah-fi-LAK-sis] a procedure for making a person insensitive to an antigen; desensitization

**antiarrhythmic drug** [an-tee-ah-RITH-mik drug] pharmacological agents that control or prevent irregular or abnormal heart rhythms

**antibiotics** [AN-tee-by-AWT-ik] category of medications that treat bacterial infections

**antibody** [AN-tih-bod-ee] proteins produced by plasma cells in response to foreign substances such as bacteria, viruses, and toxins

**anticholinergic** [AN-tee-kol-ih-NER-jik] a class of medications that antagonize actions of the parasympathetic and other cholinergic nerve fibers

**anticoagulants** [an-tee-ko-AG-yoo-lants] class of medications that delay or prevent clot formation

**anticonvulsants** [AN-tee-kon-VUL-santz] pharmacological agents that raise the seizure threshold or prevent seizure activity

**antidepressant** [AN-tee-dee-PRES-ant] medications used to improve mood and resolve depression; classes include bicyclic, tetracyclic, and monoamine oxidase (MAO) inhibitors

**antidiabetic drug** [AN-tee-dy-ah-BET-ik drug] medications that act to stabilize blood glucose metabolism by stimulation of insulin or replacement

**antidote** [AN-tee-doht] a specific agent that works to counteract a poison or its effect

**antiemetic** [AN-tee-eh-MET-ik] category of medications used to treat nausea, vomiting, and motion sickness

**antiflatulants** [an-tee-FLAT-yoo-lantz] pharmacological agents that diminish the formation of gases in the colon

**antigens** [AN-tee-jenz] substances, usually proteins, that cause the formation of antibodies and react specifically with that antibody

**antihistamines** [an-tee-HIS-tah-meenz] pharmacological agents used to counteract histamine; frequently used for allergic response

**anti-inflammatory** [AN-tee-in-FLAM-ah-toh-ree] pharmacological agents used to reduce the bodily responses without affecting the cause of inflammation

**antineoplastics** [AN-tee-nee-oh-PLAS-tiks] pharmacological agents that prevent the development and spread of neoplastic cells

**antinuclear antibodies (ANA)** [an-tee-NYOO-klee-ar AN-tih-bod-eez] immunoglobulin produced by the body that acts against its own nuclear material; indicative of autoimmune diseases such as systemic lupus erythematosus and rheumatoid arthritis

**antinuclear antibody test** [an-tee-NYOO-klee-ar AN-tih-bod-ee test] blood test used in the diagnosis of autoimmune diseases

**antioxidants** [an-tee-OX-sih-dants] substances that block or inhibit destructive oxidation reactions

**antipruritics** [an-tee-pru-RIT-iks] pharmacological agents that prevent or reduce itching

**antipsychotic** [an-tee-sigh-KAW-tik] pharmacological agents used to treat psychosis, paranoia, and schizophrenia by blocking dopamine receptors in the limbic system; also known as neuroleptics and major tranquilizers; classes include phenothiazines, high-potency agents, typical and atypical antipsychotics

**antipyretics** [AN-tee-pye-RET-iks] pharmacological agents such as aspirin and acetaminophen that reduce fever

**antisepsis** [an-tee-SEP-sis] measures taken to prevent exposure and growth of infectious agents

**antisocial personality** [AN-tee-SOH-shal per-son-AL-ih-tee] a psychiatric disorder characterized by disregard of rules, laws, morals, and ethics of society; demonstrated by lying, stealing, manipulation, and the inability to feel remorse for exploiting others

**antispasmodic** [AN-tee-spaz-MOD-ik] pharmacological agent that reduces or eliminates cramping or irregular and painful involuntary muscular contractions

**antitoxin** [AN-tee-tok-sin] serum antibody formed in response to a biological toxin that works to counteract a specific poisonous substance

**antitussives** [an-tee-TUS-ivz] pharmacological agents that suppress cough

**antrum** [AHN-trum] section of the stomach that terminates at the pylorus

**anuria** [an-YOO-ree-ah] absence of urine output or a quantity of 100 mL daily

**anus** [AYE-nus] circular, external opening of the rectum, controlled by the anal sphincter

**anxiolytic** [ANG-zee-oh-LIT-ik] pharmacological classification of drugs that relieve anxiety and stress

**aorta** [aye-OR-tah] largest artery, arises from the left ventricle

**aortalgia** [aye-or-TAL-jee-ah] pain caused by an aneurysm or other disorders of the aorta

**aortic coarctation** [aye-OR-tik ko-ark-TAY-shun] congenital narrowing of the aorta

**aortic stenosis** [aye-OR-tik ste-NOH-sis] obstruction or narrowing of the aortic valve causing significant reduction of blood flow from the left ventricle, resulting in decreased cardiac output

**aortic valve** [aye-OR-tik valv] valve located between the left ventricle and the ascending aorta

**aortoplasty** [ay-or-toh-PLAS-tee] surgical repair of the aorta

**ap-** [ap] *prefix*; separated or derived from

**apathy** [AP-ah-thee] lacking interest, indifference associated with major depression and other psychiatric conditions

**aperture** [AP-er-chur] entrance to a body cavity or channel

**apex** [AYE-pex] end point of an organ or structure

**aphagia** [ah-FAY-jee-ah] inability to swallow

**aphakia** [ah-FAY-kee-ah] condition in which the lens of the eye has been surgically removed or is absent

**aphalangia** [ah-fah-LAN-jee-ah] lacking fingers or toes

**aphasia** [ah-FAY-see-ah] condition without speech; may be defined further as expressive or receptive types

**apheresis** [aye-FER-ee-sis] a therapeutic procedure that separates out one specific type of blood cell, then reinfuses the remaining blood to the patient as a transfusion to remove harmful elements from the blood

**aphonia** [aye-FOH-nee-ah] loss of speaking voice, usually due to irritation, infection, and swelling of the larynx

**aphthous stomatitis** [AF-thus sto-mah-TYE-tis] canker sores, present as small ulcers of the oral mucosa

**apical** [AYE-pi-kul] heartbeat heard at the apex of the heart

**aplastic anemia** [aye-PLAS-tik ah-NEE-mee-ah] deficiency of blood cells resulting from failure of the bone marrow to produce adequate numbers of circulating blood cells; may be congenital or acquired

**apnea** [AP-nee-uh] cessation of respiration

**apneustic area** [ap-NEW-stik AIR-ee-uh] the brain region responsible for coordination of movements and activities essential for transition from inspiration and exhalation

**apo-** [aye-poh] *prefix*; away from

**aponeurosis** [AP-oh-nu-ROH-sis] fibrous tendon sheets that serve as attachments for muscular fibers and sometimes function as a fascia for muscles; plural is aponeuroses

**aponeurotic fibroma** [aye-poh-new-ROH-tik figh-BROH-mah] a recurrent nonmetastasizing infiltrating calcification observed most often on the palms of young patients as a small, firm nodule not attached to the dermal layer

**apoplexia** [ap-oh-PLEK-see-uh] sudden, gross bleeding in an organ; stroke caused by bleeding in the brain

**appendectomy** [ap-pen-DEK-toh-mee] surgical removal of the appendix due to infection and/or rupture

**appendiceal** [AP-en-DIH-see-al] pertaining to appendix

**appendicitis** [ah-PEN-dih-SY-tis] inflammation of the appendix with severe pain

**appendicular skeleton** [ap-PEN-dik-yoo-lar SKEL-eh-ton] the bones of the limbs and girdles attached to the axial skeleton

**appendix** [ah-PEN-diks] a thin, tubular, closed-ended section of the bowel located off the cecum that has no role in the digestive process

**apperception** [AP-per-SEP-shun] the process of clearly perceiving one's own personality

**apraxia** [aye-PRAKS-ee-ah] inability to use or manipulate objects while still being able to name and describe how the object is used

**aqueous humor** [ah-kwee-us HYOO-mor] a clear, watery fluid that is continuously probated by the ciliary processes in the posterior chamber of the eye

**-ar** [ahr] *suffix*; pertaining to

**arachnoid layer** [ah-RAK-noyd LAY-er] the middle layer of the three meninges covering the central nervous system

**arbor vitae** [AHR-bur VYE-tay] a treelike structural outline seen in the cerebellum which is visible on computerized tomography scans and other imaging studies

**-arche** [ark-ee] *suffix*; beginning or start

**areflexia** [ah-re-FLEK-see-ah] lack of reflex or response to verbal, sensory, or pain stimulation

**-arian** [ar-ee-an] *suffix*; pertaining to a person

**-aris** [ar-is] *suffix*; pertaining to

**arousal** [ah-ROWZ-ahl] component linked closely to the appearance of wakefulness and alertness

**arrector pili** [ah-REK-tor PYE-lye] muscles attached to hair follicles that cause "goose bumps" when involuntarily contracted

**arrhythmia** [ah-RITH-mee-ah] loss of regular rate or rhythm of heartbeat

**arterial blood gases** [ar-TEE-ree-al BLUD gas-ez] a laboratory study measuring the oxygen and carbon dioxide in a sample obtained from an arterial blood sample

**arterioles** [ar-TEER-ee-olz] smallest branches of arteries

**arteriopathy** [ar-TEE-ree-OP-ah-thee] collective term for disease of artery

**arteriorrhaphy** [ar-tee-ree-OR-ah-fee] suturing of an artery

**arteriorrhexis** [ar-tee-ree-oh-REK-sis] rupture of an artery

**arteriosclerosis** [ar-teer-ee-oh-skle-ROH-sis] hardening of the arteries

**arteriosclerosis obliterans** [ar-teer-ee-oh-skle-ROH-sis oh-BLIT-er-anz] a gradual narrowing of the arteries with thrombosis and degeneration of the intima

**arteriostenosis** [ar-tee-ree-oh-steh-NO-sis] narrowing of an artery

**arteriovenous fistula** [ar-teer-ee-oh-VEE-nus FIST-yoo-luh] a surgical joining of arterial and venous vessels in order to gain access to circulation during hemodialysis

**artery** [AR-tur-ee] vessel carrying blood away from the heart

**arthralgia** [ar-THRAL-gee-ah] pain in the joint from injury, inflammation, or infection

**arthrocentesis** [ar-throh-sen-TEE-sis] removal of excess fluid in a joint by inserting a needle into the joint space

**arthrodesis** [AR-throh-DEE-sis] surgical procedure to fuse the bones in a degenerate or unstable joint

**arthrogram** [AR-throh-gram] MRI, x-ray, or CT images of a joint and adjoining structures

**arthrography** [ar-THROG-ra-fee] a radiological procedure that uses a radiopaque injection into a joint that coats and outlines the bone ends and joint capsule

**arthropathy** [ar-THRO-path-ee] any disease of a joint, including inflammatory and hereditary disorders

**arthroplasty** [AR-thro-PLAS-tee] surgical replacement of a joint; often required due to degenerative joint changes

**arthroscopy** [ar-THROS-koh-pee] surgical procedure that uses a fiberoptic scope to visualize a joint and remove tissues such as damaged cartilage or bone spurs

**articular cartilage** [ar-TIK-yoo-lar KAR-tih-lij] the smooth, nonvascular, dense connective tissue that covers the end surfaces of bones forming synovial joints

**-ary** [air-ee] *suffix*; pertaining to

**asaphia** [ah-SAF-ee-ah] inability to produce clear and distinct speech

**asbestosis** [as-bes-TOH-sis] pneumoconiosis caused by inhalation of asbestosis fibers, usually from occupational exposure

**ascending colon** [ah-SEN-ding KOH-lon] segment of the bowel that extends upward on the right side of the abdomen, joining the transverse colon

**ascites** [ah-SY-teez] accumulation of excess fluid in the peritoneal cavity; most commonly caused by cirrhosis of the liver due to alcoholism, but also from heart failure and kidney disease

**-ase** [ace] or [ays] *suffix*; enzyme

**aseptic** [aye-SEP-tik] free from infectious material

**aspartate aminotransferase test (AST)** [as-PAR-tate ah-meen-oh-TRANS-fer-ace test] intracellular enzyme test to detect tissue damage in the liver, brain, and muscles

**Asperger's disorder** [AS-per-gers dis-OR-der] a developmental disorder characterized by poor social skills, repetitive behaviors, and focused interest in an esoteric topic that limits social and occupational functioning

**asphyxia** [as-FIK-see-ah] suffocation resulting from impaired or absent oxygen exchange

**aspiration** [as-pi-RAY-shun] removal of fluid or accumulation from the body by suction; inhalation of a substance or object into the airway such as food, drink, or vomitus

**aspiration pneumonia** [as-pi-RAY-shun noo-MOH-nee-ah] lung infection caused by foreign material entering the lung

**assist-control ventilation** [ah-SIST kon-TROL ven-tih-LAY-shun] mechanically supported breathing where the patient is permitted to initiate breathing but the ventilator delivers a preset volume of air and will initiate breathing if the patient's breathing slows or stops

**astasia** [ah-STA-zee-ah] inability to stand or maintain erect posture due to muscular incoordination

**asterixis** [as-ter-IK-sis] gross, involuntary, jerking tremor of the hand; also called flapping tremor

**asthenia** [as-THEE-nee-ah] lacking strength; weakness; often refers to muscular or cerebellar diseases

**-asthenia** [as-theen-ee-ah] *suffix*; weakness, decreased strength

**asthma** [AZ-mah] disease of the respiratory system characterized by increased airway irritability, narrowing and constriction of the air passages

**asthmatic** [az-MAT-ik] patient with asthma

**astrocytoma** [as-tro-sy-TOH-mah] malignant tumor of the brain or spinal cord composed of astrocytes, with typical onset in the fifth decade of life

**asymmetry** [aye-SIM-eh-tree] clinical finding of dissimilar proportion in two normally similar body parts

**asymptomatic** [AYE-simp-toh-MAT-ik] not demonstrating external signs or complaints of a disease

**asynchronous pacing** [aye-syn-KRON-us PAYS-ing] electrical stimulation of the heart that sets a rate that is independent of the heart's own pacemakers

**asynclitism** [ah-SIN-kli-tizm] presentation of the fetal head in an oblique position during labor

**asyndesis** [ah-SIN-de-sis] a brain disorder characterized by the inability to bring thoughts together to form a cohesive concept

**asyntaxia** [ah-sin-TAK-see-ah] lack of appropriate and orderly development of an embryo

**asystole** [aye-SIS-toe-lee] lack of heartbeat; cardiac standstill

**atasia** [ah-TAYZ-ee-ah] inability of the muscles of the digestive tract to relax

**ataxia** [aye-TAK-see-ah] uncoordinated muscle activity; spastic or jerky motions

**-ate** [ayte] *suffix;* pertaining to or composed of

**atelectasis** [AT-eh-LEK-tah-sis] collapse of lung tissue resulting in impaired gaseous exchange

**atherectomy** [ath-eh-REK-toh-mee] surgical removal of a fatty or lipid deposit (atheroma) in an artery

**atherosclerosis** [ATH-er-oh-skle-ROH-sis] plaque formation on the inner arterial wall of a blood vessel

**atherosclerotic plaque** [ATH-er-oh-skle-roh-tik plak] thick, hard deposit on the walls of the inner arteries that can clog the arteries in the heart and the brain or other organs

**athetosis** [ath-eh-TOH-sis] involuntary, slow, and irregular snakelike, twisting movements in the upper extremities associated with encephalitis, cerebral palsy, hepatic encephalopathy, Huntington's chorea, or drug toxicity

**-ation** [aye-shun] *suffix;* process of having or being

**-ative** [ah-tiv] *suffix;* pertaining to

**atlas** [AT-las] the first cervical vertebra (C1) located directly below the occipital bone of the cranium

**atonic bladder** [aye-TON-ik BLAD-er] inability to completely empty the urinary bladder; often associated with paralysis and diabetic neuropathy

**atony** [aye-TON-ee] lacking normal tension; flaccid or relaxed

**atopic dermatitis** [ay-TOP-ick dur-muh-TYE-tis] skin inflammation of genetic origin

**atopy** [AT-uh-pee] genetically determined

**atresia** [ah-TREE-zee-ah] absence of a normal orifice, duct, or canal such as the auditory or biliary canals

**atreto-** [ah-tret-oh] *prefix;* lack of a normally occurring opening

**atrial ectopic beats (AEB)** [AYE-tree-al ek-TOP-ik beets] early or out-of-sequence contraction of the atrium of the heart

**atrial fibrillation** [AYE-tree-al fib-ril-LAY-shun] rapid, irregular twitching of the upper chambers of the heart

**atrial septal defect** [AYE-tree-al SEP-tul DEE-fekt] an abnormal opening between the atria permitting blood to shunt back and forth

**atrioseptoplasty** [aye-tree-oh-SEP-toh-plas-tee] surgical repair of a defect in the partition between the atria of the heart

**atrioventricular canal (AV canal)** [AYE-tree-oh-ven-TRIK-yoo-lar ka-NAL] refers to a combination of defects in the atrial and ventricular septa and portions of tricuspid and mitral valves

**atrioventricular node (AV node)** [AYE-tree-oh-ven-TRIK-yoo-lar nohd] an area of specialized cardiac muscle that receives electrical impulses from the sinoatrial node and sends impulses to the ventricles, causing them to contract

**atrioventricular valve** [AYE-tree-oh-ven-TRIK-yoo-lar valv] the bicuspid (mitral) and tricuspid valves located between the atria and ventricles

**atrium** [AYE-tree-uhm] two upper heart chambers directly above the ventricles, called right and left atrium, respectively

**atrophy** [AT-roh-fee] muscle tissue wasting as a result of disuse, ischemia, or nutritional deficiencies

**attending behaviors** [at-TEND-ing BEE-hav-yehrs] nonverbal signs indicating focused listening, or interest in what another person is communicating

**attention-deficit hyperactivity disorder (ADHD)** [ah-TEN-shun DEF-eh-sit HIGH-per-ak-TIV-it-ee dis-OR-der] distractibility, short attention span, inability to follow directions, restlessness, hyperactivity, labile mood, and impulsiveness; may be caused by mild brain damage at birth, genetic factors, or other abnormalities

**attenuated vaccine** [ah-TEN-yoo-aye-ted vak-SEEN] vaccine in which the antigen's ability to produce disease has been lessened or eliminated by heat or chemical measures; after inoculation, mild symptoms may result

**-ature** [ah-tur] suffix; system composed of

**audiometry** [aw-dee-OM-eh-tree] process of measuring a patient's hearing ability

**auditory** [AW-dih-tor-ee] pertaining to hearing processes

**auditory aphasia** [AW-dih-tor-ee ah-FAY-zee-ah] impaired comprehension of spoken words in the presence of normal hearing

**auditory aura** [AW-dih-tor-ee AW-rah] abnormal sensations of sound that precede a seizure

**auditory canal** [AW-dih-tor-ee ka-NAL] opening of the external ear that leads from the external auditory meatus to the tympanic membrane

**auditory channel** [AW-dih-tor-ee CHAN-nul] transmission of messages through spoken words and cues

**auditory nerve** [AW-dih-tor-ee NERV] eighth cranial nerve; conducts impulses from the semicircular canals and the cochlea to the brain to maintain balance and the sense of hearing

**auditory ossicles** [AW-di-tor-ee OS-ih-kulz] small bones of the ear: malleus, incus, and stapes

**augmented cough** [awg-MEN-ted kawf] method of increasing force and effectiveness of chest muscles by placing the palm of the hand on the abdominal musculature below the ribs during expiration and then removing the hand during inspiration

**aural** [AW-ral] pertaining to the ear

**auricle** [AW-ri-kul] tissue and cartilage that form the C shape of the external ear and semicircular canals

**auris dexter** [AW-ris DEKS-ter] right ear

**auris sinistra** [AW-ris SIN-is-trah] left ear

**auscultation** [AWS-kul-TAY-shun] use of a stethoscope to listen to heart, lungs, and bowel sounds

**auscultatory gap** [AWS-kul-tay-tor-ee GAP] temporary disappearance of sounds at the end of Korotkoff phase I and the beginning of phase II while listening with a stethoscope

**autism** [AW-tizm] neuropsychological condition characterized by limited social and communication abilities and rigidly adhering to routines and internal thoughts

**auto-** [AW-toh] *prefix*; self

**autoimmune disorders** [aw-toh-i-MEWN dis-OR-ders] conditions in which the immune response is directed toward the self

**autologous transfusion** [aw-TOL-oh-gus trans-FYOO-shun] infusion of a previously donated unit of a patient's own blood to correct loss during surgery or other interventions

**automaticity** [aw-toh-mah-TISS-uh-tee] ability to contract without neural stimulation

**autopsy** [AW-top-see] postmortem examination to determine the cause of death

**autoregulation** [AW-toe-reg-yoo-LAY-shun] redistribution of blood flow to areas of greatest need; self-management of emotions and behavior during periods of stress

**autosomal chromosomes** [aw-toh-SOW-mal KRO-moh-sohmz] the 22 pairs of chromosomes that are responsible for characteristics other than determination of sex

**avascular** [ah-VAS-kyoo-lar] characteristic of few or no blood vessels

**aversion therapy** [ah-VUHR-shun THER-ah-pee] use of an unpleasant sensation or association to decrease destructive behaviors such as drug and alcohol abuse;

noxious stimuli may range from mild electrical shock or smells like ammonia

**axilla** [AK-sil-ah] region below the junction of the shoulder joint; armpit

**axillary lymph nodes** [AK-si-lar-ee limf nodz] lymphatic structures that collect chyme in the area below the shoulder and armpit

**axis** [AX-iss] the second cervical vertebrae (C2)

**axon** [AK-son] structural process of a nerve cell that conducts nervous impulses away from the cell body and dendrites

**AY4 antibodies** [AYE-why-for AN-tih-bod-eez] substances produced in the body that react to an antigen

**azotemia** [az-oh-tee-mee-ah] abnormal concentration of urea and nitrogenous substances in the blood caused by failure of the kidneys

# B

**B lymphocyte** [bee LIM-foh-syt] cells that are produced in the bone marrow that travel to the lymph nodes and other lymphoid tissue, becoming part of the body's immune system by producing antibodies

**Babinski sign** [bah-BIN-skee sine] extension of the great toe and abduction of the other toes when the plantar surface of the foot is stimulated; indicative of pyramidal tract involvement

**bacterial vaginosis** [bak-TEE-reh-al vaj-ih-NOH-sis] a condition caused by a disruption of normal bacterial flora in the vagina causing irritation to and drainage from the vagina

**bacteriuria** [bak-teer-ee-YOO-ree-ah] presence of bacteria in the urine; when bacterial count rises above 100,000 per mL of urine, it indicates a urinary tract infection

**bag-valve mask** [bag-valv mask] a manually operated resuscitation device used to ventilate a nonbreathing patient; the device consists of a reservoir bag, a unidirectional valve, and a face mask

**Baker's cyst** [BAY-kerz sist] a collection of fluid in the synovium of the popliteal fossa behind the knee

**balanitis** [bal-ah-NY-tis] inflammation of the skin covering the glans penis which may result from sexually transmitted diseases

**Banti's syndrome** [BAN-teez SIN-drom] condition characterized by anemia, enlarged spleen and hemorrhages, culminating in cirrhosis of the liver due to portal hypertension

**baragnosis** [bar-ag-NOH-sis] inability to estimate weight of objects, indicates presence of a parietal lobe lesion

**bariatrics** [bar-ee-AT-riks] a branch of medicine focused on treatment and management of obesity

**barium enema** [BAIR-ee-yum EN-eh-ma] infusion of radiopaque barium into the lower intestinal tract for fluoroscopic study

**barium swallow** [BAIR-ee-yum SWAL-oh] radiographic study of the phalanx and esophagus after ingestion of barium sulfate

**baroreceptor** [BAR-oh-ree-SEP-tor] nerve endings in the cardiovascular system that regulate blood pressure by responding to relative pressure within

**barotitis media** [bar-oh-TYE-tis MEE-dee-uh] middle ear inflammation caused by changes in atmospheric pressure, such as in a descending airplane or in deep-sea diving

**barotrauma** [bar-oh-TRAW-mah] damage to alveoli resulting from mechanical ventilation

**barrel chest** [BARE-el chest] an increase in the anteroposterior diameter of the chest such that it resembles a barrel rather than a normal oval shape

**Barret esophagus** [BAR-et ee-SOF-ah-gus] long-standing irritation and ulceration of the distal esophagus associated with increased risk for adenocarcinoma

**Barthel Self-Care Index** [BAHR-tel self-kare IN-deks] standardized screening tool used in older adults for measuring ability to perform self-care

**basal cell carcinoma** [BAY-sal sel kahr-si-NOH-muh] malignancy of the basal cell layer

**basal metabolic rate (BMR)** [BAY-sal met-ah-BOL-ik rayt] physiological consumption of calories as measured 12 hours after eating, sleeping, and being at complete rest

**basement membrane** [BAYS-ment MEM-brayn] a delicate noncellular layer of pliable tissue that serves as support and attachment for epithelial cells

**basophil** [BAY-soh-fil] one type of white blood cell comprising less than 1 percent of all leukocytes

**Behçet's syndrome** [BAY-sets SIN-drom] a multisystemic chronic and recurrent disease characterized by oral and genital ulcerations and uveitis of the eyes resulting in blindness

**Bell's palsy** [BELLZ PAWL-zee] temporary, peripheral, unilateral paralysis of the muscles innervated by the facial nerve that causes distorted facial expressions, ptosis, tearing, and salivation on the affected side

**belonephobia** [BEL-oh-nee-FOH-bee-ah] morbid fear of needles and other objects with sharp points

**Bence-Jones protein** [bents-jonz PRO-teenz] a protein found in urine of individuals with multiple myeloma

**Benedikt's syndrome** [BEN-eh-dikts SIN-drom] paralysis of one side of the body with spasms or tremors, and occulomotor paralysis on the opposite side

**benign** [bee-NINE] not malignant, condition of mild intensity

**benign familial polyposis** [bee-NINE fah-MIL-ee-al POL-ee-POH-sis] a hereditary condition characterized by multiple benign colonic polyps which can become malignant

**benign prostatic hypertrophy** [be-NINE proh-STAT-ik high-PER-troh-fee] enlargement of the prostate gland associated with age that is not malignant but may present obstruction of urine flow

**beryllosis** [be-ril-ee-OH-sis] pneumoconiosis caused by inhalation of beryllium salts

**beta adrenergic blocking agents** [BAY-tah ad-reh-NER-jik BLOK-ing AYE-jentz] pharmacological class of agents that occupy beta receptor sites

**beta waves** [BAY-tah wayvz] brain activity that is typical of increased neural activity

**biceps brachii** [BY-seps BRAY-kee-eye] the two muscles of the upper arm that flex the forearm and flex the hand when contracted

**biceps femoris** [BY-seps fem-OR-is] one of the posterior lateral muscles of the thigh included in the hamstring group that causes external rotation and flexion of the hip when contracted

**bicuspid** [bi-KUS-pid] having two points or parts

**bicuspid valve** [bye-KUS-pid valv] valve between the left atrium and the left ventricle; left atrioventricular valve, mitral valve

**bifurcation** [bi-fer-KAY-shun] to divide into two branches

**bigeminy** [bi-JEM-ih-nee] paired occurrences, such as heart rhythms

**bilateral** [bi-LAT-er-al] pertaining to having two sides

**bile** [BIHL] the fluid produced by the liver, stored in the gallbladder, released into the duodenum to digest fats in foods

**bile duct** [BIHL dukt] the tubular structure that bile flows through

**biliary** [BIL-ee-air-ee] pertaining to bile, gall

**biliary atresia** [BIL-ee-air-ee ah-TREE-zee-ah] congenital absence of major bile ducts; also called neonatal hepatitis

**biliary cirrhosis** [BIL-ee-air-ee sir-ROH-sis] liver disorder due to obstructed bile ducts

**biliary tract** [BIL-ee-air-ee trakt] collective term for structures involved in the delivery of bile from the liver to the duodenum; includes the gallbladder, hepatic ducts, cystic ducts, and common bile ducts

**bilirubin** [BIL-ih-ROO-bin] end product from the breakdown of old red blood cells

**bilirubin level** [BIL-ih-ROO-bin LEV-el] blood test for unconjugated, conjugated, and total bilirubin levels; levels are abnormal when there is biliary obstruction or liver disease

**biliverdin** [BIL-ih-VER-din] a greenish bile pigment; gall substance

**Billroth's I operation** [BIL-rothz wun op-er-AYE-shun] surgical removal of the pylorus and antrum of the stomach with attachment of the stomach to the duodenum; also known as gastroduodenostomy

**Billroth's II operation** [BIL-rothz too op-er-AYE-shun] surgical removal of the pylorus and antrum with closure of the ends of the stomach and duodenum, followed by attaching the stomach to the jejunum; also known as gastrojejunostomy

**bin-** [bine] *prefix*; twice or double

**bioavailability** [by-oh-ah-VAIL-ah-BIL-ih-tee] readiness of a drug to produce an effect in the circulation at the target site

**biopsy** [BY-op-see] a surgical procedure to obtain a tissue sample of a mass, tumor, or skin lesion for the purpose of cellular study

**biot respirations** [bee-OH res-pi-RAY-shunz] periods of apnea alternating with breaths of the same depth

**bipolar disorder** [by-POH-lar dis-OR-der] a mood disorder characterized by abnormally high and low moods and severe behavioral disturbance

**bladder** [BLAD-der] a saclike structure that acts as a receptacle for secretions; term generally refers to the urinary bladder

**bladder neck suspension** [BLAD-der NEK sus-PEN-shun] surgical fixation of the urethrovesical junction and the bladder neck to an elevated retropubic position to alleviate stress incontinence

**-blast** [blast] *suffix*; immature cell

**blepharitis** [BLEF-ah-RY-tis] inflammation or infection of the eyelid with redness, exudate, and scales at the bases of the eyelashes

**blepharoplasty** [BLEF-ah-roh-plas-tee] surgical revision of the eyelid

**blepharoptosis** [BLEF-ah-rop-TOH-sis] drooping of the upper eyelid tissue due to diseases that affect the muscles or nerves of the eye, such as myasthenia gravis or stroke

**blepharospasm** [BLEF-ah-roh-spazm] involuntary contraction of muscles of the eyelid

**blind spot** [BLYND spot] portion of the retina that has no ability to perceive images

**blood pressure** [BLUD presh-ur] force exerted by the circulating blood on the arterial walls at the points of contraction (diastolic) and filling (systolic)

**blood urea nitrogen** [BLUD YOO-ree-uh NIH-troh-jen] a diagnostic blood test; determines the amount of urea present in the blood that is directly related to the metabolic function of the liver and excretory function of the kidney

**blood-brain barrier** [blud-brain BAR-ee-er] selective mechanism that prevents passage of toxic or large chemicals into the brain while permitting essential substances such as oxygen and glucose to enter

**B-lymphocytes** [bee-LIM-foh-sightz] cells that produce antibodies that travel through the blood with the ability to attach to foreign cells, labeling them for destruction by phagocytes

**-body** [boh-dee] *suffix*; thing or structure

**body alignment** [BOH-dee ah-LYNE-ment] position of body parts in relation to each other or with regard to normal posture

**body dysmorphic disorder** [BOH-dee dis-MOR-fik dis-OR-der] preoccupation with minor defects in the appearance of the body, particularly the face, with the demand for frequent plastic surgery

**-bol** [bol] *suffix*; throw

**bolus** [BOH-lus] a mass of chewed food or medicine that is ready to be swallowed

**bonding** [BON-ding] formation of attachment between parent and child; adhesion of one substance to another

**bone autograft** [BOWN AW-toh-graft] procedure of using bone taken from the patient's own body to use to stabilize and fuse with bony structures

**bone densitometry** [BOWN DEN-sih-TAWM-eh-tree] refers to two types of bone density tests: dual-energy x-ray absorptiometry (DEXA) scan, and quantitative computerized topography (QCT) which determines the degree of bone mineralization

**bone marrow** [BOWN mar-row] tissue in the central cavity of long bones that functions to store fat or produce red blood cells

**bone marrow aspiration** [BOWN mar-row as-pih-RAY-shun] procedure to remove red bone marrow from the posterior iliac crest of the hipbone

**bony labyrinth** [BOWN-ee LAB-ih-rinth] a series of osseous chambers located within the temporal bone; essential to hearing

**borderline personality** [BOR-der-lyne per-soh-NAL-it-ee] a psychiatric disorder characterized by an inability to sustain stable relationships, fear of abandonment, hypersensitivity, changeable emotions, poor tolerance to stress, and overdependence

**botulism** [BOT-yoo-liz-um] illness acquired by ingesting improperly cooked or canned food containing *Clostridium botulinum*; causes paralysis and is potentially fatal

**Bowman's capsule** [BOW-manz KAP-sool] a cup-shaped structure that encloses the glomerulus in the renal tubule or nephron; also known as the glomerular capsule

**brachial artery** [BRAY-kee-ul AR-tur-ee] main blood vessel bringing blood to the arm, branching off the subclavian artery and terminating at the cubital fossa of the elbow

**brachial plexus** [BRAY-kee-ul PLEK-sus] spinal nerve network of the lower cervical and first thoracic nerves

**brachial veins** [BRAY-kee-ul vaynz] main blood vessel that returns blood from the arm, terminating at the axillary vein

**brachialis muscle** [bray-kee-AY-lis MUS-sel] muscle that flexes the forearm

**brachiocephalic** [BRAY-kee-oh-seh-FAL-ik] pertaining to the arm and head

**brachiocephalic lymph duct** [BRAY-kee-oh-seh-FAL-ik limf dukt] vessel that drains chyme from the arm

**brachiocephalic vein** [BRAY-kee-oh-seh-FAL-ik vayn] major blood vessel formed by the union of the internal jugular and subclavian veins that returns blood from the head and neck region

**brachiocyllosis** [BRAY-kee-oh-sil-OH-sis] an abnormal curvature of the arm

**brachioradialis muscle** [BRAY-kee-oh-ray-dee-AL-is MUS-sel] muscle of the lateral forearm that flexes the wrist when contracted; attached at the head of the radius

**-brachy** [bray-key] *suffix*; short

**brady-** [bray-dee] *prefix*; slow, decreased rate

**bradycardia** [bray-dee-KAR-dee-ah] abnormally slowed heart rate; less than 60 beats per minute in an adult

**bradyglossia** [bray-dee-GLOSS-ee-ah] very slow or difficult tongue movement

**bradykinesia** [bray-dee-kih-NEE-see-uh] abnormally slow movement

**bradyphrasia** [bray-dee-FRAY-zee-uh] abnormally slow speech

**bradyphrenia** [bray-dee-FREN-ee-uh] slowed thinking associated with dementia

**bradypnea** [brad-ip-NEE-uh] abnormally slow respiratory rate

**Branham's sign** [BRAN-hams sighn] compression of an arteriovenous fistula that slows the heart rate

**Braxton-Hicks contraction** [BRAKS-ton-hiks kon-TRAK-shun] irregular, nonpainful contractions occurring after the first trimester of pregnancy

**breech presentation** [breech pree-zen-TAY-shun] any position or presentation of the fetus in the pelvis other than head first

**brevicollis** [brev-ih-KOL-is] having an abnormally short neck

**bronchi** [BRONK-eye] airway passage branching off the trachea to the right and left lung fields

**bronchial asthma** [BRONK-ee-ul AZ-mah] form of airway constriction and irritability characterized by episodic dyspnea and bronchial spasm

**bronchial tree** [BRONK-ee-al tree] an anatomic complex of the trachea and bronchi

**bronchiectasis** [BRONG-kee-ek-TAY-sis] dilatation of the bronchioles due to chronic inflammatory lung disease

**bronchiectosis** [brong-kee-ek-TOH-sis] abnormal widening or dilatation of the bronchi or bronchioles as a result of inflammatory disease or obstruction

**bronchioles** [BRONG-kee-ohlz] the smaller divisions of the bronchial tree that terminate at the alveoli in the lungs

**bronchitis** [brong-KIGH-tis] an acute or chronic inflammation of the bronchial tubes

**bronchodilator** [brong-koh-dy-LAY-tor] pharmacological agent that relaxes the muscles of the bronchus, alleviating bronchospasm and increasing airflow into the lungs; used as a symptomatic treatment in conditions such as asthma

**bronchogenic pneumonia** [brong-koh-JEN-ik noo-MOH-nee-ah] acute inflammation of the bronchioles and alveoli that produces congestion

**bronchopneumonia** [BRONG-koh-noo-MOH-nee-ah] infection of the airway including the bronchi, bronchioles, and lung tissue

**bronchoscope** [BRONG-koh-skope] a small-diameter fiberoptic instrument used to visualize and biopsy the upper airway and lung tissue

**bronchospasm** [BRONG-koh-spaz-um] an involuntary, rapid contraction of the bronchiole smooth muscle

**bronchus** [BRONG-kus] section of the airway immediately posterior to the main trunk of the trachea that bifurcates into the right and left segments

**Brudzinski sign** [bryoo-JIN-skee sighn] physical finding associated with meningitis where passive flexion of the neck produces involuntary flexion of the knees and hips

**bruise** [BRUZE] bleeding into tissue

**bruit** [BROO-ee] soft blowing sound heard on auscultation, caused by turbulent blood flow

**bruxism** [BRUKS-izm] teeth-clenching or -grinding, usually occurring during sleep

**bubo** [BYOO-boh] extremely enlarged, tender lymph node of the groin that may be associated with syphilis, chancroid, or lymphogranuloma venarum

**bucca** [BUK-ah] cheek; plural is buccae

**buccal** [BUK-ahl] pertaining to the inside of the cheek

**buccal mucosa** [BUK-ahl myoo-KOS-ah] innermost surface of the facial cheek

**buccinator muscle** [BUK-si-nay-tur MUS-sel] ringlike muscle around the mouth used in smiling, compression of the cheeks, and chewing food

**bulbourethral glands** [BUL-boh-yoo-RE-thral glanz] two small, bulblike glands located on either side of the urethra just below the prostate gland that secrete a fluid component

**bulimia** [BUH-lim-ee-ah] disorder characterized by episodes of self-induced purging after binging

**bullae** [BULL-uh; BULL-ee] blister(s), or plebe(s)

**bundle branches** [BUN-del branch-ez] major conductive pathways of the heart involved in coordination of the heart muscle

**bunion** [BUN-yun] disorder of the foot associated with swelling and inflammation of the great toe; commonly seen in women who wear narrow-toed shoes

**bunionectomy** [BUN-yun-EK-toh-mee] surgical procedure to remove the prominent part of a metatarsal bone that is causing the bunion

**bursa** [BER-sah] a slender, elongated pocket of synovial membrane that contains synovial fluid and acts as a cushion to reduce friction in areas where a tendon rubs against a bone; plural is bursae

**bursectomy** [bur-SEK-toh-mee] excision of a synovial membrane containing synovial fluid located in areas where tendons pass over bones

**bursitis** [bur-SY-tis] inflammation of a fluid-filled synovial sac located over a bony prominence or point of articulation between tendon and bone

## C

**calcaneus** [kal-KAY-nee-us] the largest bone of the foot; commonly referred to as the heel

**calcitonin** [kal-si-TOH-nin] a thyroid hormone that lowers plasma calcium and phosphate ion levels by inhibiting bone resorption; increases renal excretion

**calculogenesis** [KAL-kyoo-loh-JEN-eh-sis] formation of a stone in an organ or blood vessel

**calefacient** [KAL-ee-fah-shent] to warm or to make hot, as in applying a hot compress

**calix** [KAY-liks] a cup-shaped structure within an organ, such as the kidney

**Calve-Perthes disease** [kal-VAY-PER-tas dis-EEZ] a self-limiting condition occurring in children between the ages of 2 and 12 years in which there is a necrosis of the ossification centers of bone followed by regeneration and recalcification

**canal** [kah-NAL] a narrow or tubular channel

**canal of Schlemm** [kah-NAL of shlem] space between the sclera and cornea of the eye that drains aqueous humor from the eye

**cancellous tissue** [KAN-sel-us TISH-yu] spongy or lattice-like bone formation located in the epiphyses of developing bone

**cancer** [KAN-ser] malignant, carcinoma

*Candida albicans* [KAN-dih-dah AL-bih-kanz] a gram-positive yeast organism that causes infections of the mouth, skin, and vagina

**candidiasis** [KAN-dih-DY-ah-sis] thrush; oral infection caused by the fungus *Candida albicans*, often due to immunosuppression

**capillary** [KAP-ih-lair-ee] small blood vessel connecting arteries with veins

**capitate** [KAP-ih-tayt] bone of the hand; used to describe rounded shape of structures

**carbuncle** [KAHR-bunk-ul] large furuncle

**carcinogenic** [kar-sih-noh-JEN-ik] substance, agent, or conditions that produce malignant cells

**carcinoma** [kahr-si-NOH-muh] cancerous cells; tumor or abnormal cells composed of anaplastic or abnormally shaped epithelial cells

**carcinoma in situ** [kar-si-NOH-mah in SIGH-too] malignant lesion with cellular changes but limited to the immediate tissue; precursor to invasive malignant disease

**Cardarelli's sign** [kar-da-REL-leez sighn] pulsating, lateral movement of the trachea associated with aortic aneurysm

**cardia** [KAR-dee-ah] a small area of the stomach at the point nearest the heart where the esophagus joins the stomach

**cardiac arrest** [KAR-dee-ak ah-REST] sudden stoppage of the heartbeat

**cardiac catheterization** [KAR-dee-ak kath-e-tur-i-ZAY-shun] a procedure in which a long, flexible tube is inserted into cardiac vessels via a peripheral artery or vein; images produced from the procedure can isolate vessel blockage

**cardiac conduction system** [KAR-dee-ak kon-DUK-shun SIS-tem] system of impulses guiding heart contraction comprised of the sinoatrial node, atrioventricular node, atrioventricular bundle, right atrium, right and left bundle branches, and Purkinje fibers to produce a heart contraction

**cardiac enzyme test** [KAR-dee-ak EN-zym test] battery of blood tests performed to determine the presence of cardiac damage by detecting the level of heart muscle enzymes

**cardiac notch** [KAR-dee-ak notch] anatomical landmark of the lung where the lung tissue indents to allow for the physical presence of the heart

**cardiac scan** [KAR-dee-ak skan] diagnostic study of the heart using an injection of a radioisotope and subsequent uptake by the myocardium, followed by imagery by a gamma camera of the heart beating; measures the volume of blood pumped by each ventricle

**cardiac sphincter** [KAR-dee-ak SFINK-ter] a muscular ring in the esophagus that prevents reflux of food from the stomach; also known as the lower esophageal sphincter

**cardiac syncope** [KAR-dee-ak SIN-koh-pee] transient and sudden loss of consciousness due to inadequate cardiac output associated with bradycardia, tachycardia, or myocardial infarct

**cardiac tamponade** [KAR-dee-ak tam-puh-NADE] heart compression resulting from accumulation of fluid in the pericardium

**cardiac ventricles** [KAR-dee-ak VEN-trih-klz] the two lower heart chambers directly below the atrium, called right and left ventricles, respectively

**cardioacceleratory center** [kar-dee-oh-ak-SEL-ih-rah-tor-ee SEN-ter] sympathetic nerve center that increases the heart rate and strength of contraction

**cardioinhibitory center** [kar-dee-oh-in-HIB-ih-tor-ee SEN-ter] parasympathetic nervous system area in the brain that monitors the heart rate and strength of contraction

**cardiomyopathy** [KAR-dee-oh-migh-OP-uh-thee] disease of the heart muscle or myocardium

**cardioplegia** [KAR-dee-oh-PLAY-jee-ah] deliberate and temporary paralysis of the heart for the purpose of performing surgery on the heart

**cardiopulmonary bypass** [KAR-dee-oh-PUL-mo-nair-ee BYE-pass] temporary diversion of blood circulation during heart surgery; blood passes through a heart-lung machine that receives deoxygenated blood from the venous side of circulation and then returns oxygenated blood to the patient's arterial side of circulation

**cardiorrhexis** [KAR-dee-or-reks-is] rupture of the wall of the myocardium

**cardiotonic** [KAR-dee-oh-TON-ik] exerting a favorable or enhancing effect on the heart, usually increased strength of contractions and cardiac output

**cardioversion** [KAR-dee-oh-VER-zuhn] use of electrical countershock to restore regular heart rhythm

**caries** [KAR-eez] areas of destruction of bone or dental enamel

**carina** [kah-RIH-nah] anatomical structure of a central ridge on a tissue surface

**carotid artery** [ka-ROT-id AR-ter-ee] the principal blood supply to the head and neck arising off the aortic arch

**carotid bruit** [ka-ROT-id bru-EE] systolic murmur detectable in the neck but not in the aortic area

**carotid endarterectomy** [ka-ROT-id end-ar-ter-EK-toh-mee] surgical removal of intra-arterial obstructions such as of the internal carotid artery, reducing the risk for transient ischemic attacks and strokes

**carotid pulse** [ka-ROT-id puls] systolic pulsation felt at the base of the neck

**carotid sinus syndrome** [ka-ROT-id SY-nus SIN-drom] condition where stimulation of a hyperactive carotid sinus causes a severe drop in blood pressure due to vasodilation and bradycardia resulting in syncope

**carotid transient ischemic attack** [ka-ROT-id TRANZ-ee-ent is-KEE-mik ah-TAK] ischemia of the anterior carotid arteries that lasts for 24 hours or less, causing neurological deficits in speech, vision, motor tracts, and balance

**carpal** [KAR-puhl] pertaining to wrist or carpal bones

**carpal bones** [KAR-puhl bohnz] osseous structures of the wrist, including the hemad, pisiform, triquetral, lunate, trapezium, trapezoid, capitate, and scaphoid bones

**carpal joints** [KAR-puhl joynts] articular surfaces of the wrist

**carpal tunnel syndrome** [KAR-puhl TUN-el SIN-drom] compression of the median nerve of the hand by connective tissue that causes pain, numbness, and loss of strength of the hand

**carpoptosis** [kar-pop-TOH-sis] damage to the muscles or nerves of the wrist that cause the wrist to be unable to extend

**carpus** [KAR-pus] wrist

**cartilage transplantation** [KAR-tih-lij tranz-plan-TAY-shun] surgical procedure that is an alternative to a total knee replacement; used to treat middle-aged adults with degenerative joint disease of the knee to delay the need for total knee replacement surgery

**cartilaginous** [KAR-tih-LAJ-ih-nus] pertaining to cartilage

**caruncle** [KAR-ung-kul] a small, fleshy mass

**cast** [KAST] application of a rigid form around a body part or fracture to stabilize it in a fixed position to facilitate healing

**cata-** [kat-uh] *prefix*; down

**catabolism** [ka-TAB-oh-lizm] destructive phase of metabolism

**cataplexy** [KAT-ah-plek-see] a transient episode of extreme muscular weakness, triggered by extreme emotional states such as fear, anger, or surprise; sudden and uncontrollable urge to sleep associated with narcolepsy

**cataracts** [KAT-a-rakts] clouding of the lens of the eye; treated by surgical removal and replacement with a prosthetic intraocular lens

**catastrophic reaction** [kat-ah-STROF-ik ree-AK-shun] disorganized or agitated behavior commonly associated with dementia when the individual faces overwhelming or threatening situations that are beyond his or her coping ability

**catatonic schizophrenia** [kat-ah-TAWN-ik skitz-oh-FRE-nee-ah] psychiatric disorder characterized by marked disturbance in thought process, stupor, negativism, and rigidity alternating with periods of great excitement

**categorical imperative** [KAT-ee-gor-ih-kal im-PER-ah-tiv] concept that states that clinicians should act only if the action is based on a principle that is universal

**cathartic** [ka-THAR-tic] pharmacological agents that stimulate peristalsis and evacuation of the bowel

**catheterization** [kath-e-tur-i-ZAY-shun] insertion of a flexible tube into a body cavity for the instillation or withdrawal of fluid

**cations** [KAT-eye-onz] ions with a positive charge

**cauda equina** [KAW-dah ee-KWIGH-nah] the bundle of spinal nerves arising from the lumbosacral and lumbar region

**cauda equina syndrome** [KAW-dah ee-KWIGH-nah SIN-drom] compression of nerve roots of the sacral and coccygeal nerves resulting in numbness in the buttocks, genitalia, or thigh along with disturbed bowel and bladder function

**caudal** [KAW-dal] general directional term pertaining to the tail-end or distal portion of any structure

**caudal anesthesia** [KAW-dal AN-es-thee-zee-ah] injection of a local analgesic agent into the epidural space of the sacrum

**caudal flexure** [KAW-dal FLEK-shur] bent section of the lumbosacral region of an embryo

**caus-** [kaws] *prefix;* burning

**causalgia** [kaw-SAL-jee-ah] a severe sensation of burning pain, often in an extremity

**caut-** [kawt] *prefix;* to burn

**cauterize** [KAW-ter-rize] burning tissue with thermal heat using electricity, steam, laser, or dry ice, often to destroy diseased tissue or coagulate blood vessels

**cavitis** [kay-VY-tis] inflammation of the vena cava

**cavity** [KAV-ih-tee] a hollow space in a body organ or structure; in reference to dentition, this term identifies erosion of dental structure

**cecocolopexy** [see-koh-KOH-low-pek-see] surgical fixation of the cecum

**cecum** [SEE-kum] a section of bowel located at the first portion of the large intestine that terminates at the appendix

**-cele** [seel] *suffix;* bulging or hernia

**celiac** [SEE-lee-ak] pertaining to the abdominal cavity

**celiac disease** [SEE-lee-ak dis-EEZ] malabsorption disorder caused by gluten sensitivity; celiac sprue

**celiac sprue** [SEE-lee-ak sproo] gluten enteropathy; a food allergy to the gluten in wheat that causes tissues of the small intestine to become damaged by the allergic response

**celiac trunk** [SEE-lee-ak trunk] part of the abdominal aorta from which arteries arise to take blood to the stomach, small intestine, liver, gallbladder, and pancreas

**cellular infiltration** [SEL-you-lar in-fil-TRAY-shun] movement or growth of cells from their usual location by means of unusual growth; often used to describe inflammation and some malignant neoplasms

**cellulitis** [sell-yoo-LYE-tis] inflammation of connective tissue, especially of the subcutaneous tissue

**-centesis** [sin-tee-sis] *suffix*; puncture

**central fissure** [SEN-tral FISH-ur] a central landmark depression on the surface of the liver

**central line** [SEN-tral lyne] a venous access device inserted into the subclavian vein, used to infuse medications, fluids, and other agents as well as to measure venous pressure

**cephalad** [SEF-ah-lad] toward or in the direction of the head

**cephalalgia** [SEF-al-AL-jee-ah] headache

**cephalic duct** [seh-FAL-ik dukt] channel that drains lymph from the upper chest and neck

**cephalic presentation** [seh-FAL-ik pree-zen-TAY-shun] appearance of any part of the fetal head during vaginal delivery

**cephalic vein** [seh-FAL-ik vayn] a superficial blood vessel that returns blood from the dorsal and palmar surfaces of the forearm to the subclavian vein

**-cephalus** [sef-uh-lus] *suffix*; head

**-ceps** [seps] *suffix*; head

**cerebellar gait** [sair-eh-BEL-ar gayt] a walking stance where the legs are spread widely to compensate for disruption of balance and the tendency to fall

**cerebellitis** [sair-eh-bel-EYE-tis] inflammation of the cerebellum

**cerebellum** [sair-eh-BEL-um] a large brain structure located dorsal to the pons and medulla that functions to maintain balance, ocular movement, and posture

**cerebral angiography** [SER-ee-bral an-jee-OG-ruh-fee] mapping of the cerebral blood vessels using dye and x-rays

**cerebral aqueduct** [SER-ee-bral AK-weh-dukt] a canal in the midbrain that contains cerebrospinal fluid and connects the third and fourth ventricles

**cerebral cortex** [SER-ee-bral KOR-teks] outer layer of the cerebrum

**cerebral dominance** [SER-ee-bral DOM-ih-nants] concept that one hemisphere of the brain exercises greater control or influence for functions such as speech, analytical thinking, mathematics, spatial perception, and motor control

**cerebral edema** [SER-ee-bral eh-DEE-mah] presence of increased intracranial and extracellular fluid in the white matter of the brain

**cerebral palsy** [SER-ee-bral PAWL-zee] a group of motor disorders caused by damage to motor centers of the cerebral cortex, cerebellum, or basal ganglia during fetal development, childbirth, or early infancy

**cerebral perfusion pressure** [SER-ee-bral per-FYOO-zhun PRESH-ur] force needed to ensure that adequate oxygen and nutrients are delivered to tissues

**cerebral ventricles** [SER-ee-bral VEN-trik-ulz] the four cavities within the cerebrum containing cerebrospinal fluid

**cerebrospinal fluid** [SER-eh-broh-SPY-nul FLU-id] a fluid secreted by the choroid plexuses of the ventricles of the brain, filling ventricles, subarachnoid spaces, and the spinal cord

**cerebrovascular accident** [SER-eh-broh-VAS-kyoo-lar AK-si-dent] generalized term pertaining to all strokes without regard to the underlying pathology or mechanism

**cerebrum** [SER-eh-brum] largest portion of the brain; has left and right hemispheres

**cerumen** [seh-ROO-men] waxy substance produced by glands in the external auditory meatus which functions to protect the external auditory meatus from infection by trapping microorganisms

**ceruminous glands** [se-ROO-mih-nus glanz] glands that secrete cerumen or earwax

**cervical intraepithelial neoplasia** [SER-vi-kal in-trah-ep-ih-THEE-lee-al nee-oh-PLAY-zee-ah] dysplasia of the squamous epithelium of the uterine cervix that may extend into deeper layers

**cervical nodes** [SER-vih-kal nohdz] lymph nodes located in the neck

**cervical plexus** [SER-vih-kal PLEKS-us] network of nerves in the cervical region

**cervical polyp** [SER-vih-kal POL-up] abnormal growth extending from membrane of the cervix uteri

**cervical spine** [SER-vih-kal spyn] the upper region of the neck consisting of the seven vertebrae

**cervical vertebrae** [SER-vih-kal VER-te-bray] the seven vertebral segments forming the cervical column in the region of the neck

**cervicitis** [ser-vik-SIGH-tis] inflammation of the cervix

**cervix** [SER-viks] the portion of an organ resembling a neck

**cervix uteri** [SER-viks YOO-ter-eye] the neck of the uterus through which menstrual flow and the fetus pass; structure subject to tears during delivery of a fetus

**chalazion** [kah-LAY-zee-on] a small, firm, painless lump near the edge of the eyelid, sometimes related to blockage of a meibomian gland

**chancre** [SHANG-ker] a skin ulcer associated with infection with syphilis

**chancroid** [SHANG-kroyd] a sexually transmitted infection with *Haemophilus ducreyi* that causes open, painful genital sores

**cheilectomy** [kye-LEK-toh-mee] surgical removal of osteophytes; the scraping away of bony irregularities

**cheilitis** [ky-LY-tis] inflammation and cracking of the lips and corners of the mouth due to nutritional deficiency, infection, or allergies

**cheiloplasty** [KYE-loh-PLAS-tee] surgical repair of the lip, usually because of a laceration

**cheilosis** [ky-LOH-sis] abnormal condition of the lips characterized by fissures and sores; frequently associated with vitamin B-complex deficiency

**chemosis** [kee-MO-sis] swelling of the bulbar conjunctiva of the eye that produces swelling around the cornea

**chemotaxis** [kee-mo-TAK-sis] migration of cells in response to a chemical stimulus

**chemotherapy** [kee-mo-THER-ah-pee] use of chemical agents to treat disease, especially to treat cancer

**cherry hemangioma** [CHER-ee he-man-jee-OH-mah] type of birthmark with raised, round tissue comprised of a network of blood vessels

**chest physiotherapy** [chest fiz-ee-oh-THER-ah-pee] technique of percussing or vibrating the chest wall in an effort to mobilize pulmonary secretions; usually accompanies postural drainage

**Cheyne-Stokes respirations** [CHAIN-stohks res-pi-RAY-shunz] gradual, transitory respiratory pattern characterized by rapid breathing alternating with periods of apnea, often associated with coma or impending death

**chlamydia trachomatis** [klah-MID-ee-ah trak-OH-mat-is] the causative organism responsible for sexually acquired disease in the United States

**chloasma** [kloh-AZ-mah] skin condition associated with pregnancy due to melanocyte-stimulating hormone, characterized by dark hyperpigmentation of the face and a line on the abdomen from pubis to umbilicus called linea nigra

**cholangiography** [koh-LAN-jee-AWG-rah-fee] process of recording biliary duct function with x-rays

**cholecystectomy** [koh-lee-sis-TECK-toh-mee] surgical removal of the gallbladder

**cholecystic** [KOH-lee-SIS-tik] adjective form for gallbladder, pertaining to bile

**cholecystitis** [koh-lee-sis-TIGH-tis] inflammation of the gallbladder

**cholecystogram** [koh-ee-SIS-toh-gram] radiological study of the gallbladder and bile ducts

**cholecystokinin** [KOH-lee-sis-toh-KIN-in] a hormone secreted by the jejunum, duodenum, and hypothalamus that stimulates the release of pancreatic juices and contraction of the gallbadder

**cholecystolithiasis** [koh-lee-SIS-toh-lih-THIGH-ah-sis] presence of gallstones in the gallbladder

**choledochectomy** [koh-led-oh-KEK-toh-mee] surgical incision and removal of a portion of the common bile duct

**cholelithiasis** [koh-lee-lith-AY-uh-sis] gallstones in the gallbladder or bile ducts; attack of abdominal pain caused by colonic spasms

**cholestasis** [koh-les-TAY-sis] stoppage of the flow of bile, most often due to an obstructive process

**cholesteatoma** [koh-LES-tee-ah-TOH-mah] a benign, slow-growing mass in the middle ear composed of squamous epithelium and cholesterol deposits that eventually destroys the bones of the middle ear as it invades the mastoid air cells; caused by otitis media

**cholesterol** [koh-LES-ter-ol] a component of the plasma membrane used to produce bile and steroid hormones (estrogen, progesterone, and testosterone) that can accumulate and deposit abnormally, as in atherosclerosis or gallstones

**cholinergics** [koh-lin-UR-jiks] drugs that mimic acetylcholine activity to strengthen the esophageal sphincter

**cholinesterase inhibitors** [koh-lin-ES-ter-ays in-HIB-ih-torz] pharmacological agents that prevent the breakdown of choline at the synapse; used to treat dementia

**chondrectomy** [kon-DREK-toh-mee] surgical excision of cartilage

**chondroblast** [KON-droh-blast] immature cartilage cells

**chondrodysplasia** [kon-droh-dis-PLAY-zee-uh] an inherited growth disorder of bone and cartilage that leads to skeletal malformation and dwarfism

**chondroma** [kon-DROH-mah] a benign, slow-growing tumor of cartilage

**chondrosarcoma** [kon-dro-sar-KOH-ma] malignant tumor of cartilage

**chordae tendinae** [KOR-dee TEN-di-nay] tendinous cords in the heart that look like strings attaching the papillary muscles to the cusps of the mitral and tricuspid valves

**chorion** [KOH-ree-on] embryonic membrane that makes up part of the placenta

**chorionic cavity** [koh-ree-ON-ik KAV-ih-tee] space in the extra-embryonic membrane

**chorionic villi** [koh-ree-ON-ik VIL-eye] vascular projections in the fetal membrane that become the fetal portion of the placenta

**chorioretinitis** [koh-ree-oh-ret-in-EYE-tis] inflammation of the choroid and retina of the eye

**choroid plexus** [KO-royd PLEKS-us] structures in the ventricles that secrete cerebral spinal fluid and play a role in intraventricular pressure of the brain

**Chron's disease** [KRONZ dis-EEZ] an inflammatory bowel disease involving intermittent segments of full thickness of the gastrointestinal tract, occurring most often in the terminal ileum of the small intestine or proximal large intestine; symptoms include abdominal pain, bloody diarrhea, and fistulas

**chronic** [KRAW-nik] an illness or condition with slow development and long duration, and that persists over a long period of time

**chronic obstructive pulmonary disease (COPD)** [KRAW-nik ob-STRUK-tive PUL-moe-nar-ee dis-EEZ] lung disorder caused by chronic exposure to irritants such as cigarette smoke and pollution; alveoli rupture creating large spaces and obstruction, characterized by dyspnea, severe productive cough, fatigue, and cyanosis

**chronological age** [kron-oh-LOJ-ik-al ayj] exact age of a person from birth

**chylomicrons** [ki-loh-MY-krohz] lipoproteins synthesized in the intestines that transport triglycerides to the liver

**chyme** [KIME] the semisolid mixture of digestive juices, saliva, and chewed food

**chymotrypsin** [ky-mo-TRIP-sin] an enzyme secreted by the pancreas that aids in the digestion of protein

**cicatrix** [SIK-ah-triks] scar tissue that is less elastic, often appears contracted, and lacks normal skin pigmentation

**-cidal** [sy-dal] *suffix*; to kill

**cilia** [SIL-ee-ah] small, hairlike projections on the surface of the mucosa that move in waves; singular is cilium

**ciliary body** [SIL-ee-ar-ee BOD-ee] thickened portion of the vascular tunic of the eye between the choroid and the iris

**cingulate gyrus** [SIN-gyoo-layt JY-rus] a brain structure with a long, curved convolution on the medial surface of the cortical hemisphere, continuing over the corpus callosum

**circa-** [sir-ka] *prefix*; about

**circadian rhythm** [sir-KAY-dee-ahn RITH-um] physical biorhythms affecting events including body temperature, endocrine function, and sleep cycle

**circulatory assist devices** [SUR-kyoo-lah-tor-ee ah-SIST dee-VY-sez] instruments that decrease cardiac workload and improve organ perfusion in patients with severe heart failure

**circum-** [sir-kum] *prefix*; around

**circumcision** [ser-kum-SIH-zhun] surgical removal of the foreskin or prepuce

**circumduction** [ser-kum-DUK-shun] movement in which the proximal end is fixed while the distal end moves in a circle

**circumflex artery** [SER-kum-fleks AR-tur-ee] left vessel that supplies blood to the left atrium and left ventricle

**circumoral cyanosis** [SER-kum-OR-al SY-ah-NOH-sis] bluish-gray discoloration around the mouth from abnormally low levels of oxygen and abnormally high levels of carbon dioxide in the tissues

**circumstantiality** [SER-kum-stan-she-AL-ih-tee] a disturbance in thought process evidenced by inclusion of excessive, tangential, and irrelevant information when asked a question; associated with schizophrenia and obsessive disorders

**circumvallate papillae** [ser-kum-VAL-ayt pa-PIL-aye] circular projections at the back of the tongue containing taste buds

**cirrhosis** [sir-ROH-sis] inflammation of the liver characterized by nodules and scarring; can be caused by alcoholism, viral hepatitis, or chronic obstruction of the bile ducts

**clast-** [klast] *prefix*; cell that breaks down substances

**claudication** [klaw-dih-KAY-shun] modified gait; limping

**claustrophobia** [KLAW-stroh-FOH-bee-ah] fear of enclosed or small spaces

**clavicle** [KLAV-ih-kul] a thin, rodlike bone on each side of the anterior neck; commonly referred to as the collarbone

**clavus** [KLAY-vus] thick, dry callus of skin often occurring on plantar surfaces; also known as a corn

**clavus callus** [KLAY-vus KAL-us] thickened layer of skin

**-cle** [kil] *suffix*; small

**cleft palate** [kleft PAL-at] unilateral or bilateral congenital deformity where the maxilla fails to completely close, resulting in an opening in the bone and skin

**clitoris** [KLIH-toh-ris] female external genitalia; analogous to the penis

**clitoritis** [klih-toh-RY-tis] inflammation of the external female genitalia

**CLO test (*Campylobacter*-like organism test)** [kloh test] a rapid screening test used to detect *Helicobacter pylori* by placing a biopsy of the gastric mucosa on a test pad containing urea; if present, the bacterium changes the urea to ammonia

**clonic** [KLON-ic] alternating muscular contraction and relaxation; often used to describe seizure activity

**-clonus** [klon-us] *suffix*; rapid contraction and relaxation

**closed fracture** [klosd FRAK-shur] a break in which the bone does not penetrate the overlying skin

**closed reduction** [klosd ree-DUK-shun] medical procedure in which manual manipulation of a displaced fracture is performed so that the bone ends meet to re-establish alignment

**clubbing of fingers** [KLUB-ing] increased curvature of fingertips due to long-term oxygen supply to the extremities

**coarctation of the aorta** [koh-ark-TAY-shun uv the ay-OR-tah] congenital narrowing of the aorta, often in the descending aorta near the ductus arteriosus

**-coccus** [kaw-kus] *suffix*; spherical bacterium

**coccygeal** [kok-SIJ-ee-al] pertaining to the tailbone or coccyx

**coccygeal plexus** [kok-SIJ-ee-al PLEK-sus] spinal nerve network in the coccyx region

**coccyx** [KAWK-siks] tailbone; a group of several small, fused vertebrae that are not individually numbered

**cochlea** [KOK-lee-ah] a coiled structure located in the inner ear that is shaped like a snail shell and contains the organ of corti

**cochlear duct** [KOK-lee-ar DUKT] a membranous space inside the cochlea that surrounds the organ of corti

**cochlear implant** [KOK-lee-ar IM-plant] an amplification device that is surgically inserted into the cochlea in which wires are placed through the round window and into the cochlea

**cochleopalpebral reflex** [KOK-lee-oh-PAL-peh-bral REE-fleks] contraction of the obicularis palpebrarum muscle in response to sudden loud noise

**cognition** [kog-NIH-shun] intellectual ability to think including language, calculation, memory, reasoning, and social skill; tested by various neurocognitive screening tools for dementia, depression, and other brain disorders

**cognitive-behavioral therapy** [KOG-nih-tiv-bee-HAY-vyer-al THAIR-ah-pee] a form of psychotherapy based on the premise that beliefs, attitudes, and thought patterns are learned and can be modified, using various techniques such as guided imagery and self-talk to produce desirable emotions

**cogwheel rigidity** [KOG-weel ri-JID-ih-tee] stiff, jerky movements of the muscles as if clicking in a gear; associated with Parkinson's disease and side effects of neuroleptic medications

**coitus** [KO-ih-tus] sexual intercourse

**colitis** [ko-LYE-tis] an inflammatory condition of the large intestine

**collagen** [KOL-uh-jen] fibrous protein

**collateral ligaments** [koh-LAT-er-al LIG-ah-ments] tough, fibrous tissues that provide lateral and medial stability to the knee, ankle, and elbow joints

**Colles fracture** [KOL-eez FRAK-shur] displacement of the distal end of the radius and ulna

**-collis** [kol-is] *suffix*; condition of the neck

**colloid bath** [KOL-oyd bath] immersion in water with dissolved soothing agents to treat skin disorders such as puritis

**collum** [KOL-um] necklike structure between the head and shoulder

**colocolostomy** [koh-low-koh-LOS-toe-mee] surgical creation of a new opening between two segments of the colon

**colon** [KOH-lon] section of the large intestine comprised of the ascending colon, transverse colon, descending colon, and sigmoid colon

**colonic** [koh-LON-ik] pertaining to the colon

**colonic polyposis** [ko-LON-ik pol-ee-POE-sis] an inherited condition where large numbers of pendulous growths develop in the mucosa of the colon, with near-certain development of colon cancer; treatment is prophylactic colectomy

**colorectal adenocarcinoma** [KOH-loh-REK-tal AD-eh-no-KAR-sih-NO-mah] cancerous tumor of the colon caused by colonic polyps or ulcerative colitis that becomes cancerous

**colostomy** [koh-LOS-toh-mee] surgical creation of an artificial anus on the abdominal wall

**colostrum** [koh-LOS-trum] liquid that contains protective antibodies secreted by the mammary glands for the few days immediately following childbirth

**colpoperineoplasty** [KOL-poh-per-ih-NEE-oh-plas-tee] surgical reconstruction of the vagina and perineum

**colposcopy** [kol-POS-koh-pee] visual examination of the vagina and cervix using an optical magnifying instrument called a colposcope

**coma** [KO-mah] state of unconsciousness in which the patient cannot be aroused, even with powerful stimuli; may result from trauma, disease, or toxicity

**comedo** [KOM-ee-doh] accumulation of sebum and keratin in the opening of a hair follicle

**comminuted fracture** [COM-mih-nyoo-ted FRAK-shur] disruption of the integrity of bone by the bone being crushed into several pieces

**commissurotomy** [KOM-ih-shur-OT-oh-mee] surgical division of a heart valve due to ventricular hypertrophy

**common bile duct** [KOM-mon BIHL dukt] the duct formed by the juncture of the cystic and hepatic ducts

**communicable** [koh-MYOON-ih-kah-bul] capable of being transferred or transmitted to another individual

**compound fracture** [KOM-pownd FRAK-shur] disruption of the integrity of bone in which the bone breaks through the overlying tissue

**compression fracture** [com-PRESH-un FRAK-shur] a bone break, especially in a short bone, that disrupts osseous tissue and collapses the affected bone

**computerized axial tomography (CAT, CT scan)** [kom-PYOO-ter-ized AK-see-al toh-MOG-rah-fee] a radiological procedure that uses x-rays to create images of successive slices of the body and its organs

**con-** [kon] *prefix*; together or with

**conchae** [CONG-kay] the three elongated, bony projections known as the superior, middle, and inferior turbinates or nasal conchae; singular is concha

**concussion** [kon-KUSH-un] brain trauma resulting in transient and/or immediate loss of consciousness due to injury to the soft structure of the brain

**condom catheter** [CON-dom KATH-eh-ter] an externally applied urinary collection device applied directly to the penis for the management of urinary incontinence

**conduction system** [kon-DUK-shun SYS-tem] the electrical system of the heart consisting of specialized muscle cells in the right atrium that initiate electrical impulses that spread throughout the heart, causing it to contract

**conductive hearing loss** [kon-DUK-tiv HEER-ing loss] decreased auditory function caused by a lesion or obstruction of the outer ear

**conductive keratoplasty (CK)** [kon-DUK-tiv KER-ah-toh-PLAS-tee] surgical procedure to correct farsightedness using heat to shrink tissues around the edge of the cornea to resolve the refractive error

**condyle** [KON-dyle] articular surface with rounded shape at the end of a bone

**condyloid joints** [KON-di-loid JOYNTS] articular surfaces in which the oval surface of one bone fits into the elliptical surface of another

**condyloma acuminatum** [kon-dih-LOH-ma ah-ku-mih-NAH-tum] genital wart due to sexually transmitted disease; plural is condyloma acuminata

**cone cells** [KOHN sells] cells in the retina of the eye that are sensitive only to color; there are three types of cones: those that respond to red light, those that respond to green light, and those that respond to blue light

**congenital** [con-JEN-ih-tal] present at birth

**congenital dislocation of the hip** [con-JEN-ih-tal dis-loh-KAY-shun uv thuh HIP] poor or incomplete formation of the ligaments or acetabulum causing the hip to be loose and not properly functioning

**congestive heart failure** [kon-JES-tiv hart FAYL-yer] disease in which the heart muscle cannot keep pace to provide the body with oxygenated blood

**conjugate gaze** [CON-joo-gayt GAYZ] both eyes move together as a unit

**conjunctiva** [kon-junk-TY-vah] mucous membrane surrounding the eyeball and posterior surfaces of the eyelids; plural is conjunctivae

**conjunctivitis** [kon-JUNK-tih-VY-tis] inflamed, reddened, and swollen conjunctivae with dilated blood vessels; it has a variety of causes, including foreign substance in the eye, mechanical irritation, or dryness

**conjunctivitis, bacterial** [kon-JUNK-tih-VY-tis, bak-TEER-ee-al] inflammation and redness of the mucous membrane of the anterior eyeball from bacterial infection; commonly referred to as "pinkeye"

**conscious sedation** [KON-shus see-DAY-shun] a medically controlled state of depressed consciousness during which the client retains the ability to maintain a continuously patent airway and to respond appropriately to physical stimulation or verbal commands

**constipation** [CON-stih-PAY-shun] failure to have regular, soft bowel movements

**contact dermatitis** [KON-takt dur-mah-TYE-tis] skin inflammation caused by an irritant coming in contact with the skin

**continuous passive motion machine (CPM)** [kon-TIN-yoo-uhs PAS-iv MOH-shun ma-SHEEN] device that increases range of motion and stimulates healing of the articular cartilage by decreasing swelling and the formation of adhesions

**continuous positive airway pressure (CPAP)** [kon-TIN-yoo-uhs POZ-ih-tiv AIR-way PRESH-ur] a method of keeping the airway open using increased air pressure delivered by a nasal or face mask to treat obstructive sleep apnea, acute pulmonary edema, and congestive heart failure

**contra-** [kon-tra] *prefix;* opposing or against

**contracture** [kon-TRAK-chur] condition of fixed resistance to the passive stretch of a muscle; associated with paralysis or lack of use of a muscle group

**contraindication** [KON-trah-in-dih-KAY-shun] term used in pharmacology to refer a disease or condition that makes the use of certain drugs harmful to the patient

**contralateral** [kon-trah-LAT-er-al] directional term, pertaining to the opposite side of the body

**controlled mandatory ventilation** [kon-TROLD MAN-dih-tor-ee ven-tih-LAY-shun] use of a machine to replace and override any impulse to breathe in an intubated patient

**contusion** [con-TEW-zhun] bruise, bleeding into tissue

**convergence** [con-VER-jens] medical procedure testing the ability of both eyes to turn medially by holding up an index finger and moving it progressively closer to the patient's nose to test the function of the medial rectus muscles; maximum convergence is called the near point

**conversion** [con-VER-shun] neurological, sensory, or motor deficits that occur without physical basis; there may be sudden blindness, deafness, paralysis, or inability to speak

**convoluted tubule** [CON-voh-LEW-ted TOOB-yool] small, twisting tubule in glomerulus in the kidney that connects Bowman's capsule and the loop of Henle

**convolutions** [kon-voh-LEW-shunz] folds separated by depressions

**convulsion** [kon-VUL-shun] seizure with a series of sudden, involuntary contractions of muscles of the face, trunk, and extremities

**coprolalia** [kop-roh-LAY-lee-ah] involuntary verbalizations or gestures that are socially inappropriate, vulgar, obscene, or racist due to Tourette's syndrome

**cor pulmonale** [KOR pul-mo-NAL-ee] heart disease characterized by right ventricular hypertrophy due to lung disease

**coracoid process** [KOR-ah-koyd PROS-ess] a small projection that resembles a bent finger; is a point of attachment for several muscles of the arm and chest

**cordate** [KOR-dayt] having the shape of a heart; can be used to describe heart-shaped tumors

**corium** [KOH-ree-um] area of skin immediately below the epidermis; also known as dermis

**cornea** [KOR-nee-ah] the transparent anterior portion of the sclera of the eye

**corneal abrasion** [KOR-nee-ahl ah-BRAY-shun] loss of or damage to superficial layers of the cornea due to trauma or repetitive irritation, such as a foreign particle under a contact lens

**corneal reflex** [KOR-nee-al REE-fleks] closing of the eyelid in response to stimulation of the cornea of the eye

**corneal transplant** [KOR-nee-al TRANZ-plant] grafting a donated cornea to restore function of the eye

**corneal ulcer** [KOR-nee-al UL-ser] chronic arterial infection and sloughing off of necrotic tissue

**coronal plane** [kor-OH-nal PLAYN] pertaining to the vertical division of the body into front and back sections

**coronary artery disease** [KOR-oh-nar-ee AR-ter-ee dis-EEZ] condition in which the myocardium receives inadequate blood supply, pertaining to the heart

**coronary bypass** [KOR-oh-nar-ee BYE-pass] surgical shunting of heart blood vessels around areas of blockage to restore supply to the heart muscle

**coronary circulation** [KOR-oh-nar-ee sir-ku-LAY-shun] blood supply to the heart tissue

**coronary sinus** [KOR-oh-nar-ee SYE-nus] vascular channel draining the coronary veins into the right atrium

**corpora cavernosa** [COR-por-ah kav-er-NOH-sah] spongy erectile tissues within the penis or clitoris that become engorged during sexual excitation; singular is corpora cavernosum

**corpus callosum** [KOR-pus kuh-LOH-sum] a broad band of white matter connecting the cerebral hemispheres

**corpus spongiosum** [KOR-pus spun-jee-OH-sum] erectile tissue that becomes engorged with blood during sexual arousal, causing the penis to become firm and erect; this tissue is located along the underside of the penis

**corrugator muscle** [KOR-yoo-gay-tor MUS-sel] a facial muscle that draws the eyebrows together to frown

**cortex** [KOR-teks] the outermost layer of any organ such as a lymph node, kidney, ovary, thymus, or cerebrum

**cortical bone** [KOR-tih-kal bohn] a superficial, thin layer of compact bone; also called substantia corticalis

**cortisol** [KOR-ti-sol] hydrocortisone secreted by the adrenal cortex

**coryza** [ko-RI-za] inflammation of nasal passages associated with profuse nasal discharge, as seen with the common cold

**costochondral joint** [KOS-toh-KON-dral JOYNT] the area where the costal cartilage meets the bone of the rib

**cough** [KAWF] forceful exhalation with the intent of clearing the airway of food, fluids, or mucus

**counterirritant** [kown-ter-IR-ih-tant] a topically applied agent that produces an inflammatory reaction for the purpose of distraction from a primary sensation, usually pain in deeper tissues

**coup-contre coup** [koo-kon-trah KOO] brain injury with damage occurring on side of impact and on the opposite side of impact due to the forward and backward motion of the brain within the skull

**coxa magna** [KOK-sah MAG-nah] enlargement of the femoral head causing osteoarthritis of the joint

**coxa valga** [KOK-sah VAL-gah] deformity of the angle of the femoral neck resulting in outward displacement

**coxalgia** [kok-SAL-jee-ah] pain in the hip joint

**coxarthrosis** [koks-ar-THRHO-sis] pain and inflammation of the hip joint due to arthritis

**cradle cap** [KRAY-del kap] seborrheic dermatitis in infants

**cranial** [KRAY-nee-al] pertaining to the skull or head

**cranial bones** [KRAY-nee-al bohnz] osseous structure of the head including the frontal, parietal, temporal, occipital, sphenoid, ethmoid, nasal, vomer, and lacrimal bones, and the inferior nasal concha

**cranial nerves** [KRAY-nee-al nervs] the twelve paired nerves that emerge from or enter the brain; I: olfactory, II: optic, III: oculomotor, IV: trochlear, V: trigeminal, VI: abducens, VII: facial, VIII: vestibulocochlear, IX: glossopharyngeal, X: vagus, XI: accessory, and XII: hypoglossal

**craniectomy** [kray-nee-ECK-toh-mee] surgical procedure of opening the skull and removing a portion of the bone

**craniosynostosis** [KRAY-nee-oh-sin-os-TOH-sis] premature closing of the cranial sutures during the first 18 months of life

**cranium** [KRAY-nee-um] bony structure that contains the brain

**creatinine** [kree-AT-in-in] a substance in urine that is found in elevated quantities in patients with muscular dystrophy and other pathologies

**Credé method** [kre-DAY METH-od] use of external pressure to compress the bladder and express urine when nervous impulses are interrupted

**crepitus** [KREP-ih-tus] crunching or grinding sounds produced in certain pathological states such as severe arthritis or pneumonia

**cretinism** [KREE-tin-izm] congenital hypothyroidism that can cause mental retardation if left untreated

**Creutzfeldt-Jakob disease** [KROITZ-felt-YAH-kop dis-EEZ] progressive fatal neurological disorder caused by an infectious protein particle contracted from cows infected with bovine spongiform encephalopathy

**-crine** [kreen] *suffix;* secretion of a substance

**Crohn's disease (CD)** [KROHNZ dis-EEZ] inflammatory bowel disease that can involve any part of the digestive tract; most often found in the ileum, resulting in obstruction of the intestine

**cross-section** [KROSS-sek-shun] to cut across a plane to study tissue or cells

**croup** [KROOP] laryngotracheobronchitis in infants and young children caused by bacterial or viral infection of the pharynx in children, characterized by difficult and noisy respiration and a hoarse cough

**crusts** [KRUSTZ] hard coverings that result when exudate on the skin dries

**cry-** [kry] *prefix;* cold

**cryosurgery** [krye-oh-SIR-jir-ee] localized freezing of diseased tissues for surgical removal

**cryotherapy** [kry-oh-THAIR-ah-pee] use of cold in the treatment of a disease or injury

**cryptorchidism** [krip-TOR-kih-dizm] failure of one or both testicles to descend

**cryptosporidiosis** [KRIP-toh-spoh-rid-ee-OH-sis] infection with the protozoa from the genus *Cryptosporidium* that is transmitted through exposure to contaminated food or may be sexually transmitted; typical symptoms are severe diarrhea and abdominal cramps

**cuboid** [KYOO-boyd] one of the seven bones of the ankle

**culdocentesis** [kul-doh-sen-TEE-sis] surgical puncture to remove fluid from the cul-de-sac of Douglas

**-cule** [kule] *suffix*; pertaining to small size

**Cullen's sign** [KU-lens sine] bluish discoloration around the umbilicus in postoperative clients; can indicate intro-abdominal or perineal bleeding

**culture and sensitivity** [KUL-chur and SEN-sih-HIV-ih-tee] a laboratory test that utilizes a swab of material from a body part or wound to grow bacteria in culture medium in a Petri dish to identify the infectious agent, then determine which antibiotics are capable of impeding their growth

**cuneiform** [kyoo-NEE-ih-form] wedge-shaped bones of the hand

**curettage** [kuu-reh-TAHZH] surgical procedure in which tissue is scraped away using a curette

**Cushing's syndrome** [KOOSH-ings SIN-drom] a metabolic disorder resulting from the chronic and excessive production of cortisol by the adrenal cortex

**Cushing's triad** [KOOSH-ings TRY-ad] response associated with increased intracranial pressure or compromised circulation in the brain stem; characterized by hypertension, increased systolic pressure with widened pulse pressure, bradycardia, and irregular respirations

**-cusis** [kyoo-sis] *suffix*; hearing

**-cuspid** [kus-pid] *suffix*; points or projections

**cutaneous** [kyoo-TAY-nee-us] pertaining to or involving the skin

**cutaneous papillomas** [kyoo-TAY-nee-us pah-pil-OH-mahz] skin tags

**cuticle** [KEW-ti-kul] fold of skin at the nail root; eponychium

**cyan-** [sigh-an] *prefix*; blue in color; lacking oxygen

**cyanosis** [sigh-ah-NOH-sis] bluish skin and mucous membranes resulting from a lack of oxygen in the blood

**cycl-** [sy-kl] *prefix*; circular; cycle

**cycloplegia** [sigh-kloh-PLEE-jee-ah] loss of functionality of the ciliary muscle of the eye due to denervation or medication

**cyclothymia** [sigh-kloh-THY-mee-ah] chronic, mild bipolar disorder in which the patient demonstrates mild mood swings with periods of symptom-free intervals for several months

**cyst-** [syst] *prefix*; pertaining to the urinary bladder or sac

**cystic duct** [SIS-tik dukt] the duct through which bile from the gallbladder passes into the common bile duct

**cystic fibrosis** [SIS-tik figh-BROH-sis] an inherited disorder characterized by excessive, thick mucus which causes obstructions in the respiratory and gastrointestinal tract

**cystitis** [sis-TYE-tis] inflammation of the urinary bladder and ureters resulting from bacterial infection, tumor, or calculus

**cystocele** [SIS-toh-seel] herniation or protrusion of the urinary bladder into the vagina

**cystoplasty** [SIS-toh-plas-tee] any reconstructive surgical procedure on the urinary bladder

**cystoscopy** [sis-TOS-koh-pee] process of visual examination of the urinary bladder using a fiberoptic scope

**cystostomy** [sis-TOS-toh-mee] creation of a new opening into the urinary bladder for drainage

**cystotomy** [sis-TOT-oh-mee] incision into the urinary bladder

**-cyte** [syte] *suffix*; pertaining to a cell

**cytology** [sy-TOL-oh-jee] study of cells

**cytolysis** [sy-TOL-ih-sis] destruction of living cells

**cytomegalovirus** [SY-toh-MEG-ah-loh-VY-rus] a beta-group herpes virus that may be transmitted through sexual or intimate contact that may cause permanent disability, including hearing loss and mental retardation for infants and blindness and mental disorders for adults

**cytophotocoagulation** [SY-toh-foh-toh-koh-AG-yoo-LAY-shun] destruction of a portion of the ciliary body using an intense beam of light from a laser

**cytosol** [SY-toh-sol] the liquid portion within the cell membrane

**cytotoxic** [sigh-toh-TAWK-sik] pharmacological agents or other substances known to be detrimental or destructive to cells

**cytotoxin** [sigh-toh-TOK-sin] an antibody or other substance that attacks the cells, preventing their normal function and/or destroying them

**cyturia** [sigh-TUR-ee-ah] presence of any type of cells in the urine

# D

**dacry-** [dak-ree] *prefix*; pertaining to tears

**dacryocystitis** [DAK-ree-oh-sis-TY-tis] infection of the lacrimal sac of the eye

**dacryocystorhinostomy** [DAK-ree-oh-SIS-toh-ry-NAWS-toh-mee] surgical procedure that creates a new opening between the lacrimal sac and nose

**dacryorrhea** [dak-ree-oh-REE-ah] excessive flow of tears; possible causes include inflammation or infection of the eye

**dacryostenosis** [dak-ree-oh-sten-OH-sis] narrowing of the lacrimal duct due to cysts, tumors, or stone formation

**dactyl** [DAK-til] a single finger or toe

**de-** [dee] *prefix*; reversal of, absence

**de Lange's syndrome** [dee-LANJ SIN-drom] congenital disorder characterized by mental retardation, small head, small stature, generalized failure to thrive, and hirsutism

**debridement** [day-breed-MOWN] removal of necrotic tissue to foster the regeneration of healthy tissue

**decerebrate posturing** [dee-SER-eh-brayt POS-chur-ing] physical presentation of rigid extension of the trunk, arms, hands, legs, and feet; associated with lesions of the brain stem

**decerebrate rigidity** [dee-SER-ee-brayt ri-JID-ih-tee] particular body position caused by a lesion of the upper brain stem; characterized by rigid extension of limbs, internal rotation of the arms, and notable plantar flexion of the feet

**decibel (dB)** [DES-ih-bel] the intensity of a sound or tone; measurement noted on audiograms and other assessments of hearing

**decorticate posturing** [dee-KOR-tih-kayt POS-chur-ing] physical sign of pathology in the corticospinal tracts characterized by flexion of the arms and legs

**decubitus ulcers** [dee-KEW-bit-us UL-surz] pressure sores

**deep tendon reflex** [deep TEN-don REE-fleks] neurological response to percussion of tendons which produces muscular contraction as demonstrated by the patellar and Achilles reflexes

**deep vein thrombosis** [deep vayn throm-BOH-sis] blood-clot formation in a deep vein, occurring most frequently in the iliac and femoral veins

**defecation** [DEF-eh-KAY-shun] process of elimination of end products of digestion by bowel movement

**defibrillation** [dee-fib-ri-LAY-shun] administration of electrical shock to restore cardiac muscle conduction and contractions

**defibrillator** [dee-FIB-rih-lay-tor] a medical device that delivers an electric shock to the atria or ventricles of the heart to restore normal heart rhythm; may be an internal or external device

**degenerative** [dee-JEN-er-ah-tiv] progressive destruction of cells due to disease or aging process

**degenerative joint disease (DJD)** [dee-JEN-er-ah-tiv JOYNT dis-EEZ] loss of articular cartilage due to aging and cumulative injury to a joint

**deglutition** [DEE-gloo-TISH-un] the process of swallowing and/or passing food, liquid, or air

**dehiscence** [dee-HIS-enss] bursting open or splitting of tissue along a natural or sutured line

**dehydration** [dee-hy-DRAY-shun] state of body water deficit

**deleterious** [del-ee-TER-ee-us] actions causing injury, harm, or destruction to a patient

**delirium** [deh-LEER-ee-um] acute confusion, disorientation, and agitation due to toxic levels of body chemicals, drugs, or alcohol in the blood that affect the brain

**delirium tremens** [deh-LEER-ee-um TREM-enz] caused by withdrawal symptoms from alcoholic intoxication; includes restlessness, tremors of the hands, hallucinations, sweating, and increased heart rate and seizures

**delta rhythm** [DEL-tah RITH-um] wave pattern on an electroencephalogram typical of deep sleep

**delta wave** [DEL-tah wayv] premature upstroke of the initial polarization of the heart; a complex of an electrocardiogram finding associated with an atrioventricular bypass tract

**deltoid muscle** [DEL-toyd MUS-sel] muscle that abducts the upper arm

**delusion** [dee-LOO-zhun] a fixed false belief that is sustained even when provided evidence to the contrary; due to psychosis or delirium

**delusional disorder** [dee-LOO-zhun-al dis-OR-der] a psychotic state wherein the patient experiences continued false beliefs despite the efforts of others to persuade or the evidence showing otherwise

**dementia** [dee-MEN-shee-ah] loss of cognitive and intellectual functioning due to a variety of brain disorders

**demineralization** [dee-MIN-er-al-ih-ZAY-shun] reduction of minerals such as calcium in body tissues, particularly related to bone

**dendrites** [DEN-rites] branched nerve fibers carrying impulses toward the cell body

**-dendron** [den-dron] *suffix*; the branched portion of a nerve cell that receives an impulse

**dens** [DENZ] a toothlike projection from the second cervical vertebra (C2), upon which the head rotates

**deontology** [dee-ohn-TOL-oh-jee] a system of ethical decision making that considers the intrinsic moral significance of an action as the basis of decisions

**deoxygenated** [dee-OKS-eh-jen-aye-ted] without sufficient oxygen

**deoxyhemoglobin** [dee-OKS-ee-HEE-moh-glo-bin] hemoglobin that is lacking oxygen

**depersonalization** [dee-PER-son-al-ih-ZAY-shun] loss of connection (dissociative process) between personal thoughts and a sense of self and the environment in which the client reports feeling that he/she is in a dream or watching a movie of him/herself, and things feel unreal and strange; viewing or treating an individual as an object rather than as a person

**depigmentation** [dee-PIG-men-TAY-shun] white patches of skin due to loss of melanocytes

**depolarization** [dee-POE-lar-ih-ZAY-shun] the reduction of the membrane potential in nerve or muscle cells to a less negative value

**depressed fracture** [dee-PREST FRAK-shur] disruption of the cranium where bone is pushed inward toward the brain

**depression** [dee-PRESH-un] pervasive alteration in mood characterized by low mood, feelings of sadness, social withdrawal, psychomotor retardation, sleep disorder, despair, hopelessness, helplessness, and suicidal thoughts

**-derma** [derm-uh] *suffix*; skin

**dermabrasion** [DERM-ah-bray-zhun] dermatological procedure that mechanically scrapes away skin layers

**dermagraphism** [der-mah-GRAF-izm] condition where hives are produced by scratches or touching the skin

**dermatitis** [DER-mah-TYE-tis] skin inflammation from any source

**dermatoautoplasty** [der-mah-toh-AW-toh-plas-tee] skin graft of tissue taken from another area of the patient's body

**dermatology** [der-mah-TOL-oh-jee] study or treatment of the skin

**dermatome** [DER-mah-tome] area of skin supplied by a sensory nerve

**dermatomyositis** [DER-mah-toh-migh-oh-SIGH-tis] inflammation of skin and muscles

**dermatophyte** [der-MAH-toh-fite] fungal agent that infects the skin, hair, and nails

**dermatophytoses** [DER-mah-toh-figh-TOH-seez] skin infections caused by fungi

**dermis** [DER-mis] layer of skin below the epidermis

**descending colon** [dee-SEN-ding KOH-lon] segment of the small intestine posterior to the splenic flexure and before the sigmoid colon

**desensitization** [dee-sen-si-ti-ZAY-shun] procedure for making a person insensitive to an antigen; antianaphylaxis

**-desis** [dee-sis] *suffix*; binding, fuse together

**desquamation** [des-kwa-MAY-shun] shedding of skin; exfoliation

**detrusor muscle** [dee-TRU-sor MUS-sel] smooth muscle of the bladder wall

**DEXA scan (dual-energy x-ray absorptiometry scan)** [DEK-sah scan] a radiological procedure that measures bone mineral density to determine if demineralization from osteoporosis has occurred

**dextroscoliosis** [DEKS-troh-skoh-lee-OH-sis] an abnormal, excessive, C- or S-shaped lateral curvature of the spine

**di-** [dye] *prefix*; two

**dia-** [dy-ah] *prefix*; through, throughout, or completely

**diabetes insipidus** [dye-ah-BEE-teez in-SIP-ih-dus] chronic pituitary disorder causing antiduretic hormone (ADH) insufficiency

**diabetes mellitus** [dye-ah-BEE-teez mel-EYE-tus] a metabolic disorder characterized by decreased use of carbohydrates and increased proteins and lipids due to absence of insulin production

**diabetes mellitus, type I** [dye-ah-BEE-teez mel-EYE-tus] juvenile diabetes characterized by destruction of insulin producing beta cells of the islets of Langerhans in the pancreas; possible etiologies include genetic inheritance and viral infection that triggers an autoimmune response

**diabetes mellitus, type II** [dye-ah-BEE-teez mel-EYE-tus] condition in which the body produces insufficient insulin, or defective use of insulin produced; treatment includes oral agents, insulin if needed, dietary restriction, and weight loss

**diabetic ketoacidosis (DKA)** [DYE-ah-BET-ik KEE-toh-AS-ih-DOH-sis] in uncontrolled diabetes and starvation, an abnormal utilization of carbohydrates results in excessive production of ketone bodies during oxidation of fatty acids

**diabetic neuropathy** [DYE-ah-BET-ik nyoo-ROP-ah-thee] damage to peripheral nerves of the lower legs and feet due to poorly controlled blood glucose levels

**diabetic retinopathy** [DYE-ah-BET-ik ret-ih-NAWP-ah-thee] condition associated with long-standing diabetes; characterized by damage to the retina of the eye by interrupted vascularization from hemorrhages, micro-aneurysms, and waxy deposits

**diagnosis** [dye-ag-NOE-sis] identification of a pathological state or disorder

**dialysis** [dye-AL-ih-sis] artificial procedure used to replace normal kidney filtering by using an external filtration system

**diaphoresis** [dye-uh-foh-REE-sis] profuse sweating

**diaphragm** [DYE-ah-fram] a curved, muscular membrane that divides the thoracic and abdominal cavities

**diaphysis** [dy-AF-ih-sis] the midsection or shaft of a long cylindrical bone, such as the femur

**diarrhea** [DYE-ah-REE-uh] abnormally frequent and loose, watery stools with increased peristalsis caused by an infection (bacteria, viruses), irritable bowel syndrome, ulcerative colitis, lactose intolerance, or a drug side effect

**diastole** [dye-AS-toh-lee] relaxation of the heart, allowing it to refill with blood for the next contraction

**diastolic blood pressure** [dye-us-TOL-ik BLUD presh-ur] force exerted by the circulating blood on the arterial walls during ventricular relaxation and filling

**diathermy** [DYE-ah-therm-ee] therapeutic use of electromagnetic ultrasound waves to heat muscle tissue

**diencephalon** [dye-en-CEF-uh-lon] brain structure containing the thalamus and hypothalamus

**diffusion** [di-FYOO-zhun] movement of molecules in a solution or a gas from an area of high concentration to one of low concentration

**digital subtraction angiography** [DIJ-ih-tahl sub-TRAK-shun an-jee-OGH-rah-fee] computerized imaging of the vasculature with visualization on a monitor screen following the intravenous injection of iodine through a catheter

**digitalis** [dij-ih-TAL-is] a pharmacological agent that increases the strength of heart muscle contraction

**digitalization** [dij-ih-tal-ih-ZAY-shun] administration of a larger loading dose of digitalis to speed therapeutic response without producing toxic symptoms

**dilated funduscopy** [DIH-layt-ed fun-DOS-kohp-ee] procedure to examine the posterior cavity using mydriatic eyedrops to dilate the pupil (a process known as cycloplegia)

**dilation and curettage** [dye-LAY-shun and kuh-reh-TAJH] dilation of the cervix and scraping of the endometrium

**dilation and extraction** [dye-LAY-shun and eks-TRAK-shun] dilation of the cervix and removal of the products of conception

**diplegia** [di-PLEE-jee-ah] paralysis involving both arms or both legs

**diplococcus** [dip-loh-KOK-us] spherical or oval-shaped bacterium, occurring in pairs; plural is diplococci

**diplopia** [dih-PLOH-pee-ah] visual disturbance where single objects are perceived as two objects; caused by increased intracranial pressure or by multiple sclerosis that affects nerve conduction

**-dipsia** [dip-see-uh] *suffix*; thirst

**dis-** [dys] *prefix*; away from

**disc** [DISK] small, circular bone with two flat surfaces; acts as a cushion to decrease impact during body movements

**discoid lupus erythematosus** [DYS-koid LOO-pus er-ih-thee-mah-TOH-sus] autoimmune disease of connective tissue

**dislocation** [dis-loh-KAY-shun] displacement of the end of a bone from its normal position within a joint; usually caused by injury or trauma

**dismember** [dis-MEM-ber] to remove an arm or leg by surgical amputation

**disorganized schizophrenia** [dis-OR-gan-izd skitz-oh-FRE-nee-ah] a severe thought disorder characterized by incoherent thought processes, inappropriate affect, silly and childlike mannerisms, but without delusions

**disorientation** [DIS-ore-ee-en-TAY-shun] loss of information as to person, date, time, surroundings, and situation; caused by acute illness or dementia

**displaced fracture** [dis-PLAYSD FRAK-chur] when broken bone ends are pulled out of their normal anatomical alignment

**dissecting aneurysm** [dys-SEK-ting AN-yoo-riz-um] bulge or tear occurring between the arterial walls due to blood forcing its way through a tear in the intima between the arterial layers

**dissection** [dih-SEK-shun] surgical removal or extensive incision

**disseminated** [dih-SEM-ih-nay-ted] condition of wide dispersement throughout an tissue, organ, or body part

**disseminated intravascular coagulation** [dih-SEM-ih-nay-ted IN-tra-VAS-kyoo-lar koh-ag-yoo-LAY-shun] disruption of clotting due to hyperstimulation of coagulation pathways resulting in unfocused clotting action that exhausts necessary clotting factors such that generalized and severe bleeding occurs

**dissociated nystagmus** [dih-SOH-see-ayt-ed nis-TAG-mus] rhythmic movements of the eyes where the movements differ in directions, rate, and severity

**dissociative fugue** [dih-SOH-see-ah-tiv FEWG] impulsive flight from one's life and familiar surroundings following a traumatic event; the patient begins a new life in a new location and functions normally without recall of the past

**dissolution** [dih-soh-LEW-shun] rate at which a drug becomes a solution

**dista equinus** [DIS-tah ek-QWEE-nus] limited ability to dorsiflex the foot; associated with clubfoot

**distal** [DYS-tal] away from the center or point of origin

**distal interphalangeal joint (DIP)** [DYS-tal in-ter-fah-LAN-jee-ahl joynt] the articular surface between the last two phalanges in a finger or toe

**distribution** [dis-tri-BYOO-shun] movement of drugs from the blood into various body liquids and tissues

**distributive shock** [dis-TRIB-yoo-tiv shok] abnormal pooling of blood in the extremities due to anaphylaxis, sepsis, or spinal cord injury

**diuresis** [dye-yoo-REE-sis] increased urine formation and secretion

**diuretics** [dye-yoo-RET-iks] pharmacological agents that increase urinary output

**diurnal** [dy-YUR-nal] pertaining to a daily occurrence of body rhythms, such as circadian rhythm

**diverticulitis** [DYE-ver-TIK-yoo-LYE-tis] feces become trapped inside a diverticular sac, resulting in inflammation and infection, abdominal pain, and fever

**diverticulosis** [dy-ver-tik-yoo-LOH-sis] formation of pouches in the wall of the colon, usually without inflammation

**diverticulum** [DYE-ver-TIK-yoo-lum] area of the intestinal surface where the mucosa has been forced out through small defects in the wall of the colon

**divulsor** [dih-VUL-sor] a medical tool used to dilate a body part, such as the urethra

**dopamine** [DOHP-ah-meen] neurotransmitter in the brain

**Doppler** [DOP-lur] determination of blood flow; velocity, direction, and possible occlusion using a transducer placed over the blood vessel; data obtained is analyzed by computer for pathology

**dorsal** [DOR-sal] pertaining to back part

**dorsal column** [DOR-sal KOL-lum] white matter in the posterior region of the spinal cord that contains motor neurons

**dorsal horn** [DOR-sal horn] horn-shaped projection of gray matter in the posterior region of the spinal cord

**dorsal muscles** [DOR-sal MUS-selz] skeletal muscles of the back including the trapezius and latissimus dorsi

**dorsal ramus** [DOR-sal RAY-mus] branch of spinal nerves that passes on the back surface to innervate skin, muscle, and bones of the vertebral column

**dorsal recumbent** [DOR-sal rih-KUM-bent] position of a patient lying down on the back, with the face up

**dorsal reflex** [DOR-sal REE-fleks] involuntary contraction of the muscles of the back in response to irritation of the skin over the erector spinae muscles

**dorsal root** [DOR-sal root] sensory nerve fibers of the spinal cord

**dorsal root ganglion** [DOR-sal root GANG-lee-on] a mass of nerve tissue containing the cell bodies of sensory neurons that is located on the dorsal surface of the nerve root

**dorsalis pedis** [dor-SAL-is PEE-dis] pulse found on the top surface of the foot

**dorsiflexion** [dor-si-FLEK-shun] movement of a body part in toward the center and upward

**dorsodynia** [dor-soh-DIN-ee-ah] pain in the upper muscles of the back

**-dose** [dohs] *suffix*; measured quantity or amount

**-drome** [drohm] *suffix*; running

**duct** [DUKT] an open channel through which secretions or other substances pass

**ductus arteriosus** [DUK-tus ar-TEER-ee-OH-sus] an oval opening in the septum between the atria in the heart that exists before birth and closes at birth, when breathing begins

**ductus deferens** [DUK-tus DEF-er-enz] a long, narrow tube that receives spermatozoa from the epididymis; also known as the vas deferens

**dumping syndrome** [DUMP-ing SIN-drom] physical effects of rapid gastric motility following gastric surgery; these effects include diaphoresis, tachycardia, the urge to lie down, diarrhea, and dehydration in severe cases; relieved by frequent small meals without liquids

**duodenal** [DOO-OD-eh-nal] pertaining to the duodenum

**duodenocholangitis** [dyoo-OD-en-oh-koh-lan-JYE-tis] inflammation of the duodenum and common bile duct

**duodenorrhaphy** [dyoo-oh-deh-NOR-ah-fee] suturing of the duodenum

**duodenum** [DOO-oh-den-um] a 10-inch-long section of bowel that immediately follows the stomach and connects with the jejunum

**dura mater** [DYOO-rah MAH-ter] the tough, fibrous membrane that forms the outermost covering of the central nervous system

**dyad** [DIE-ad] a pair, or two people in an interaction; often used to describe a mother-and-newborn interaction

**-dynia** [dye-nee-ah] *suffix*; painful

**dys-** [dis] *prefix*; faulty, painful, difficult, or abnormal

**dysarthria** [dis-AR-three-uh] difficulty forming clear speech due to dysfunction of the throat muscles

**dysboulia** [dis-BYOO-lee-ah] difficulty focusing on a task; poor concentration or thinking ability

**dyschromia** [dys-KROH-mee-uh] abnormal color of skin due to disease, radiotherapy, or cytotoxic drugs

**dysconjugate** [dis-CON-joo-gayt] condition in which the eyes do not move in tandem

**dyscrasia** [dis-KRAY-zee-ah] blood-related diseases affecting blood cells or platelets

**dysentery** [DIS-en-tair-ee] bacterial infection caused by an unusual strain of *E. coli* bacterium in the large intestine; symptoms include watery diarrhea mixed with blood and mucus

**dysesthesia** [dys-es-THEE-zee-uh] perception of an irritating sensation in response to normal stimuli due to nerve dysfunction

**dyskinesia** [dis-ki-NEE-zee-ah] experiencing difficulty in performance of voluntary movements

**dyslogia** [dis-LOH-jee-ah] impaired speech and reasoning due to a mental disorder

**dysmenorrhea** [dys-men-oh-REE-ah] painful menstruation

**dyspareunia** [dis-pah-RYOO-nee-uh] painful sexual intercourse

**dyspepsia** [dis-PEP-see-ah] indigestion or epigastric pain that may be accompanied by gas or nausea; possibly caused by excess secretion of stomach acid, overeating, spicy foods, or stress

**dysphagia** [dis-FAY-jee-ah] difficulty swallowing

**dysphonia** [dis-FOH-nee-ah] difficulty producing speech with regard to sound quality and pronunciation

**dysphoria** [dis-FOR-ee-ah] generally unhappy mood, depression, and anxiety

**dysplasia** [dis-PLAY-zee-ah] abnormal growth and development of tissue

**dyspnea** [disp-NEE-uh] difficulty breathing or shortness of breath

**dysrhythmia** [dis-RITH-mee-ah] irregular heart rhythm, rate, or sequence of cardiac activation

**dysthymia** [dis-THY-mee-ah] chronic, mild to moderate depression

**dystocia** [dis-TOE-see-ah] difficult childbirth due to large fetal size, small pelvic outlet, or malpositioning of the fetus, such as breech presentation

**dystonia** [dis-TOH-nee-ah] state of hyper- or hypotonicity of tissue; most often used in reference to muscle tone

**dysuria** [dis-YOO-ree-ah] pain during urination, often caused by infection, irritation, or obstruction of the urinary tract

# E

**e-** [ee] *prefix*; without, absent; away from or outside

**-eal** [eel] *suffix*; pertaining to

**ec-** [ek] *prefix*; out or away from

**ecchymosis** [EK-ih-MOH-sis] large hemorrhages or bruises on the skin

**eccrine** [EK-rin] denoting the flow of sweat

**echocardiogram** [ek-oh-KAHR-dee-oh-gram] image of the heart produced by ultrasound

**echogenic** [ek-oh-JEN-ik] characteristic of body tissues that resonate echoes of sound which are captured under ultrasound examination

**echolalia** [EK-oh-LAY-lee-ah] disorder of speech associated with schizophrenia where the patient automatically repeats (echoes) what someone else has said

**-ectasis** [ek-tay-sis] *suffix*; dilation or expansion

**ecto-** [ek-toh] *prefix*; outside

**ectogenous** [ek-TOJ-eh-nus] conditions produced from sources outside of the body; disease that is caused by events outside the body such as infections or traumatic injury

**-ectomy** [ek-toh-mee] *suffix*; to cut, excise, or remove

**ectopic** [ek-TOP-ik] malplacement of an organ or an object; for example, an ectopic pregnancy, which occurs outside of the uterus—or an event such as a heartbeat

**ectropion** [ek-TROH-pee-on] weakening of connective tissue in the lower eyelid in older patients causing the eyelid to turn outward, exposing the conjunctiva and causing dryness and chronic conjunctivitis

**eczema** [EK-ze-mah] genetic inflammatory skin disorder

**edema** [eh-DEE-mah] swelling of a body part

**edentulous** [ee-DEN-tyoo-lus] lacking natural teeth

**efferent** [EF-er-ent] conduction or activity moving outward

**efferent lymphatic vessel** [EF-er-ent lym-FAT-ik VES-sel] a structure that carries lymph toward the periphery

**efferent nerve** [EF-er-ent nerv] a peripheral nerve that conveys impulses from the central nervous system to the peripheral nerves; opposite of an afferent nerve

**effusion** [ee-FYOO-zhun] accumulation of fluid

**egesta** [ee-JEST-ah] the unabsorbed food fragments that are passed through the digestive tract

**ejaculation** [ee-JAK-yoo-LAY-shun] series of contractions producing emission of 2–5 mL of semen from the male urethra

**ejaculatory** [ee-JAK-yoo-lah-tor-ree] pertaining to the emission of semen from the male urethra

**ejaculatory duct** [ee-JAK-yoo-la-tor-ee dukt] the passage formed by the junction of the duct of the seminal vesicles and ductus deferens through which semen enters the urethra

**ejection fraction** [ee-JEK-shun FRAK-shun] the percentage of blood emptied from the ventricle during contraction; normal value for healthy hearts is 60–70 percent but may be much lower with valve disorders or myocardial infarction

**ejection murmur** [ee-JEK-shun MUR-mur] an abnormal cardiac sound produced by pumping of blood into the aorta or pulmonary arteries that stops prior to the closure of the aortic or pulmonic valves

**elasticity** [ee-las-TIS-ih-tee] demonstrating the ability to stretch

**electroanalgesia** [ee-lek-troh-an-al-JEE-zee-ah] use of electrical stimulation to compete with pain stimuli for transmission to the spinal cord; may be delivered through the skin or by an implantable device

**electrocardiogram** [ee-lek-troh-KAHR-dee-oh-gram] record of the electrical forces producing heart contractions

**electrocochleography** [ee-LEK-troh-kok-lee-OG-rah-fee] process of recording the electrical activities of the cochlea of the inner ear

**electroconvulsive therapy (ECT)** [ee-LEK-troh-con-VUL-siv THAIR-ah-pee] use of electrical current and electrodes on the head to produce seizures while sedated; alters the brain chemistry to treat severe depression more rapidly than antidepressant drugs

**electroencephalogram** [ee-LEK-troh-en-SEF-ah-loh-grahm] graphic recording of the brain's electrical activity

**electroencephalograph** [ee-LEK-troh-en-SEF-ah-loh-graf] an instrument used to record the electrical activity of the brain

**electrolarynx** [ee-LEK-troh-LAR-inks] an external device applied to the throat to amplify breath sounds in patients following surgical removal of the larynx

**electrolysis** [ee-lek-TROL-ih-sis] destruction of tissue by electric current

**electrolytes** [ee-LEK-troh-lites] soluble, inorganic ions, such as sodium and chloride, found in body fluids

**electromyography** [ee-LEK-troh-migh-OG-rah-fee] record of muscular activity for diagnostic purposes using electrodes

**electron** [ee-LEK-tron] a negatively charged subatomic particle

**electrophoresis** [ee-LEK-troh-for-EE-sis] movement of particles within an electric field toward a cathode or anode

**elephantiasis** [el-eh-fan-TYE-ah-sis] massive swelling of the lower extremities or genitalia; also called pachydermas

**elimination** [ee-LIM-ih-nay-shun] process of removal of undigested and residual liquids from the body

**elytro-** [el-eye-troh] *prefix*; pertaining to the vagina

**emaciation** [ee-may-see-AY-shun] excessive leanness earned by muscle wasting

**embolectomy** [em-boh-LEK-toh-mee] removal of a clot from a blood vessel by surgical or enzymatic methods

**embolism** [EM-boe-lizm] mass of undissolved matter present in a blood or lymphatic vessel brought there by the blood or lymph current

**embolization** [em-bol-ih-ZAY-shun] formation and release of a substance to occlude blood vessels in the treatment or prevention of hemorrhaging

**embolotherapy** [em-boh-loh-THAIR-ah-pee] intentional obstruction of the lumen of a blood vessel by injection of a solution or dislodgement of thrombus or plaque

**embolus** [EM-bow-lus] substance or mass that stops the flow of a vessel

**embryology** [em-bree-OL-oh-jee] study of the origin and development of a fetus from fertilization up to the time of birth

**embryonic stage** [em-bree-ON-ik STAJ] developmental stage that occurs during the first 2–8 weeks after fertilization of a human egg

**emesis** [EM-eh-sis] expelled food or chyme

**-emesis** [em-ee-sis] *suffix*; vomiting

**emetic** [ee-MET-ik] an agent that causes vomiting

**-emia** [ee-muh] *suffix*; blood condition

**-emic** [ee-mik] *suffix*; pertaining to the blood or substance in blood

**emmetropia** [em-eh-TRO-pee-ah] normal vision

**emphysema** [em-fih-SEE-mah] chronic and irreversible damage to alveoli characterized by trapped air in the lung; productive cough, often due to smoking or pollution

**empyema** [em-pye-EE-mah] presence of pus in a bodily cavity; used most often in reference to pyothorax

**emulsification** [ee-MUL-si-fi-kay-shun] process of breaking down large globules of fats into smaller particles

**en-** [en] *prefix*; in

**-ence** [ens] *suffix*; state of

**encephalitis** [en-sef-ah-LYE-tis] inflammation of the brain due to bacterial or viral infection

**encephalocele** [en-SEF-ah-loh-seel] protrusion or herniation of the brain and meninges

**encephalomalacia** [en-SEF-ah-loh-mah-LAY-sha] softening of the brain due to ischemia or infarction

**encephalomyelopathy** [en-SEF-ah-loh-mye-LOH-path-ee] disease that affects both the brain and spinal cord

**encephalopathy** [en-sef-ah-LOP-ah-thee] cerebral dysfunction due to an insult to the brain such as a toxin, injury, inflammation, or anoxic event

**encephalosclerosis** [en-SEF-ah-loh-skle-ROH-sis] hardening of the brain, especially the cerebrum, due to plaque formation or hypertension

**encopresis** [en-koh-PREE-sis] repeated passage of stool into the clothing in a child older than age five in the absence of gastrointestinal illness or disability

**end-** [end] *prefix*; within or inside

**endarterectomy** [end-art-er-EK-toh-mee] surgical excision of fatty deposits along with diseased endothelium and significant portions of the arterial lining

**endo-** [en-doh] *prefix*; within or inside

**endocardium** [en-doh-KAR-dee-um] the lining of the heart chambers

**endocrine system** [EN-doh-krin SIS-tem] structures within the body that are capable of secreting hormones; includes the hypothalamus, pituitary gland, thyroid gland, pancreas, testis, ovaries, adrenal glands, thymus, parathyroid glands, and pineal gland

**endocrinology** [EN-doh-krin-OL-oh-jee] the study of the endocrine system

**endogenous** [en-DOJ-eh-nus] disease that originates from factors inside the body; for example, autoimmune disorders

**endolymph** [EN-doh-lymf] liquid within the membranous labyrinth of the inner ear

**endometriosis** [en-doh-mee-tree-OH-sis] presence of endometrial tissue at sites other than the uterus

**endometritis** [en-doh-mee-TRY-tis] inflammation of the endometrium (lining of the uterus) due to bacterial infection

**endometrium** [en-doh-MEE-tree-um] the innermost layer of the uterine wall

**endomysium** [en-doh-MYZ-ee-um] the sheath of connective tissue that surrounds each muscle fiber

**endoneurium** [en-doh-NOO-ree-um] connective tissue surrounding an individual nerve fiber

**endopericarditis** [EN-doh-per-ee-kar-DY-tis] inflammation of the endocardium and pericardium of the heart

**endoplasm** [EN-doh-plazm] the portion of the cell between the cell membrane and nucleus that contains the cellular organelles

**endoplasmic reticulum** [en-doh-PLAS-mik reh-TIK-yoo-lum] a network of microscopic channels or tubes extending throughout the cytoplasm that serves as a transport system for materials within the cell

**endoscope** [EN-doh-skope] an instrument used to examine the interior of the body

**endoscopic retrograde cholangiopancreatography** [en-doh-SKOP-ik RET-roh-grade ko-LAN-jee-oh-pan-KREE-ah-toh-grah-fee] use of a fiberoptic scope to examine the pancreatic, bile, and hepatic ducts followed by injection of a contrast medium for radiography of the biliary and pancreatic ducts

**endotoxin** [en-doh-TOK-sin] a poisonous substance in the walls of gram-negative bacteria that produces a systemic inflammatory response and sepsis

**endotracheal** [EN-doh-TRAY-kee-al] pertaining to the innermost aspect of the trachea

**endotracheal intubation** [en-doe-TRAY-kee-al in-tyoo-BAY-shun] passage of a tube into the trachea through the nose or mouth to open the airway for delivery of air, oxygen, or anesthesia

**end-stage renal disease** [end-stayj REE-nal dis-EEZ] final phase of kidney disease marked by the inability to filter the body's blood

**-ent** [ent] *suffix*; person or agent

**enteral nutrition** [EN-ter-ahl nu-TRI-shun] delivery of nutrients through a gastrointestinal tube or other artificial means

**enterobiasis** [en-ter-oh-BY-ah-sis] pinworm infestation of the large intestine

**enterocolectomy** [EN-ter-oh-koh-LEK-toh-mee] surgical excision of the terminal ileum, cecum, and ascending colon

**enterocolitis** [EN-ter-oh-koh-LY-tis] inflammation of the small bowel due to bacterial or viral infection; possible causative agents include rotaviruses, *Campylobacter*, *Escherichia coli*, and *Salmonella* bacterial species

**enterospasm** [EN-ter-oh-SPAZM] sudden, involuntary, painful contraction of intestinal muscles

**enterotomy** [en-ter-OT-oh-mee] surgical incision into the small intestine

**-entery** [en-ter-ee] *suffix*; condition of the intestine

**entodynia** [en-toh-DYE-nee-ah] intestinal pain

**entropion** [en-TROH-pee-on] weakening of the muscle in the lower eyelid, occurring most often in older adults

**enucleation** [ee-nyoo-klee-AYE-shun] surgical procedure to remove the entire structure of the eye from the orbit due to trauma or a tumor

**enuresis** [en-yoo-REE-sis] involuntary nighttime bed-wetting, particularly in children

**environmental disease** [en-VY-rawn-MEN-tal dis-EEZ] illness associated with or due to external substances

**enzyme** [EN-zime] chemical substance produced by the body's endocrine system or organs to break down large molecules into smaller components for digestion; often ends with the *suffix* -ase

**ependymoma** [ep-en-dye-MOH-mah] brain neoplasm tumor derived from ependymal cells

**epi-** [ep-ih] *prefix*; upon, surface, or above

**epicardium** [ep-ih-KAHR-dee-um] outer heart layer; membranous lining of the inner heart

**epicondylitis** [EP-ih-kon-dih-LY-tis] inflammation of the elbow joint at the point of the articular surfaces of the humerus

**epicranius muscle** [ep-ee-KRAY-nee-us MUS-sel] muscle that raises eyebrows, as demonstrated by the expression of surprise

**epidemic** [ep-ih-DEM-ik] occurrence of a disease in greater-than-expected proportion over a geographic region

**epidemiology** [EP-ih-dee-mee-OL-oh-jee] study of the distribution and determinants of health-related states or events in populations

**epidermis** [ep-ih-DER-mis] outermost, superficial skin layer

**epidermolysis** [ep-ih-DER-moh-LIE-sis] separation of the dermal and epidermal layers of skin

**epididymis** [ep-ih-DID-ih-mis] a long, coiled duct that carries sperm from the seminiferous tubules of the testes to the vas deferens

**epididymitis** [EP-ih-did-ih-mye-tis] acute or chronic inflammation of the epididymis resulting from a variety of conditions, including urinary tract infection, venereal disease, prostatitis, or prolonged use of indwelling urinary catheters

**epididymoorchitis** [ep-ih-di-dye-MOOR-ky-tis] inflammation of the testes and the epididymis

**epigastric** [EP-ih-GAS-trik] abdominal region between the tip of the sternum and above the umbilicus

**epigastric tamponade** [EP-ih-GAS-trik tam-pon-AYD] insertion of a tampon or plug in the epigastric region to control bleeding

**epiglottic** [EP-ih-GLOT-ik] pertaining to the epiglottis

**epiglottis** [EP-ih-GLOT-is] a valvelike structure in the throat that seals off the larynx or airway, shunting food, saliva, and other liquids into the esophagus

**epiglottitis** [EP-ih-glot-TYE-tis] severe infection or inflammation of the epiglottis and surrounding tissues which can result in stridor, respiratory distress, and partial to complete airway obstruction; occurs most commonly in children ages 2–12

**epihyal** [ep-ih-HIE-yal] pertaining to the arch of the hyoid bone at the base of the tongue

**epilepsy** [EP-ih-lep-see] disorder affecting the central nervous system; characterized by recurrent seizures

**epinephrine** [ep-ih-NEF-rin] adrenal medulla hormone; adrenaline

**epineurium** [ep-ih-NEW-ree-um] connective tissue around a nerve trunk

**epiphyseal line** [ee-PIF-ih-seel lyn] the closed border of the growth plate at the end of a bone when it has stopped growing

**epiphyseal plate** [eh-PIF-ih-seel playt] a disc of cartilage located between the epiphysis and the metaphysis of long bones during growth

**epiphysis** [ee-PIF-ih-sis] the bulbous portion of bone located at the proximal and distal ends of long bones; plural is epiphyses

**epiphysis cerebri** [eh-PIF-ih-sis SER-eh-brye] pineal gland; a cone-shaped organ in the brain that secretes melatonin

**episiorrhaphy** [eh-piz-ee-OR-ah-fee] suturing of the vulva and perineum

**episiotomy** [eh-piz-ee-OT-oh-mee] process of cutting the vulva; used to assist delivery of the fetus

**epispadias** [ep-ih-SPAY-dee-us] congenital defect in which the urethral opening is located on the penis dorsum in males and the clitoris in females

**epithelial root** [ep-ih-THEE-lee-al root] nail part beneath the cuticle

**epithelium** [ep-ih-THEE-lee-um] cellular layer that forms the epidermis of the skin and outermost surface of the serous mucous membranes

**eponychium** [ep-OH-nik-ee-um] fold of skin near the nail root

**equi-** [ek-wee] *prefix*; equal, as in size or distance

**equianalgesic** [EK-wah-an-al-JEE-sik] the amount of a drug required, whether administered orally or parenterally, needed to produce the same analgesic effect when changing from one formulation to another

**equivocal** [ee-QUIV-oh-kul] questionable, doubtful, or vague

**Erb palsy** [erb PAWL-zee] paralysis of the upper arm and shoulder due to a lesion of the upper trunk of the brachial plexus or the fifth and sixth cervical roots

**erector spinae muscles** [ee-REK-tor SPY-nee MUS-selz] muscular group of the dorsal spine that originates at the sacrum, ilium, and lumbar vertebrae and attaches at the ribs and upper thoracic vertebra; the function is to maintain upright posture and extend the vertebral column

**erotomania** [ER-oh-toh-MA-nee-ah] pathological preoccupation with erotic ideas and behavior; delusional belief that the patient is romantically involved with a celebrity or desirable person; associated with acute mania and schizophrenia

**erysipelas** [er-ih-SIP-ee-las] acute cellulitis of the skin

**erythema** [er-ih-THEE-ma] redness on the skin

**erythroblastosis fetalis** [eh-RITH-row-blas-TOW-sis fee-TAL-is] hemolytic disorder of a newborn characterized by jaundice, anemia, generalized edema, and enlargement of the spleen and liver

**erythrocytosis** [eh-RITH-roh-sye-TOE-sis] abnormally increased amount of red blood cells in circulation; associated with hypoxemia and polycythemia vera

**erythropoiesis** [eh-RITH-roh-poy-EE-sis] production of red blood cells

**erythropoietin** [eh-rith-roh-POY-eh-tin] a glycoprotein hormone released into the bloodstream in response to hypoxia which increases the production of red blood cells; also a hormone secreted by the kidney that stimulates the bone marrow to produce red blood cells

**eschar** [ES-kar] thick scar that forms over a healed burn

**Escherich's reflex** [ESH-er-iks REE-fleks] involuntary muscular contraction of the mouth when the mucosa of the lips is stimulated; this is noted particularly in newborns

**-esis** [ee-sis] *suffix*; condition or state of being

**esophageal** [ee-SOF-ah-JEE-al] pertaining to the esophagus

**esophageal sphincter** [ee-SOF-ah-JEE-al SFINK-ter] valve at the end of the esophagus as it joins with the stomach that prevents reflux of gastric contents into the esophagus

**esophageal varices** [ee-SOF-ah-JEE-al VAR-ih-seez] twisted, swollen veins in the esophagus

**esophagitis** [ee-SOF-ah-JY-tis] chronic inflammation of the esophagus; this inflammation can progress to esophageal ulcers or cancer of the esophagus

**esophagospasm** [ee-SOF-ah-goh-spazm] sudden, involuntary, often painful contraction of the muscles of the esophagus

**esophagus** [ee-SOF-ah-gus] a flexible, muscular tube leading from the pharynx to the stomach

**esotropia** [es-oh-TROH-pee-ah] turning inward of the eyeball

**esterase** [ES-ter-ace] an enzyme that splits organic compounds such as fats

**estra-** [es-trah] *prefix*; outside of

**estradiol** [es-trah-DEE-ohl] a naturally occurring estrogen that is formed by the ovary, placenta, testes, and adrenal cortex

**estrogen** [ES-troh-jen] hormones secreted by the placenta, and in small amounts by the adrenal cortex; responsible for many female reproductive functions, including secondary female characteristics

**ethmoid bone** [ETH-moyd bohn] bone forming the anterior base of the cranium, bony nasal septum, and medial walls of the eye sockets

**ethmoid sinuses** [ETH-moyd SIGH-nus-ez] one of the air chambers within the ethmoid bone

**etiology** [ee-tee-AWL-oh-jee] underlying cause of a disorder

**eu-** [yoo] *prefix*; normal or good

**eucrasia** [yoo-KRA-see-ah] state of normal health with balance in all activities or processes

**eupnea** [YOOP-nee-ah] breathing with normal depth and rate

**eury-** [yur-ee] *prefix*; broad or thickened

**eustachian tube** [yoo-STAY-shun toob] a small canal between the inner ear and throat that allows air pressure in the middle ear to equalize with air pressure in the mouth and outside the body

**eustress** [YOO-stress] a type of stress that results in positive change or growth

**eutocia** [yoo-TOE-see-uh] normal labor

**eversion** [ee-VER-shun] turning a body part outward

**Ewing's sarcoma** [YOO-ingz sar-KOH-mah] a malignancy of the bones of the extremities and shoulder girdle, with a typical onset before age 20

**ex-** [eks] *prefix*; out or away from, external

**exacerbation** [eks-az-er-BAY-shun] increase in symptoms or severity of disease

**excisional biopsy** [ek-SIH-zhun-al BY-op-see] removal of an entire suspected lesion for microscopic examination

**excoriation** [eks-koh-ree-AY-shun] skin abrasion

**excrete** [eks-KREET] to move substances produced within endogenous tissues and organs out of the body

**excretory cystogram** [EKS-cree-tor-ee SIS-toh-gram] a radiographic examination of excretory organs

**excretory urogram** [EKS-cree-tor-ee YOO-roh-gram] radiographic images of an injected dye as it is processed and eliminated by the kidney

**exercise stress test** [EKS-er-zyz STRES test] a cardiac assessment that determines heart rate, blood pressure, and electrocardiography (ECG) while exercising at various intensities, usually on a treadmill

**exercise-induced asthma** [EKS-er-zyz-in-DOOST AZ-mah] a subtype of asthma where bronchoconstriction and dyspnea are triggered by physical exertion

**exercise-induced urticaria** [EKS-er-zyz-in-DOOST ur-tih-KAR-ee-uh] large, red, raised lesions of the skin resulting from histamine release during exercise

**exhalation** [eks-ha-LAY-shun] the process of pushing air out of the lungs

**exo-** [eks-oh] *prefix*; outside, external

**exogenous** [eks-OH-jeh-nus] originating outside an organ or body part

**exophthalmos** [eks-off-THAL-mohs] outward bulging of the anterior surface of the eye with a startled, staring expression; when presentation is unilateral, etiology is often a tumor behind the eye, but when presentation is bilateral, the patient usually has hyperthyroidism

**exotoxin** [eks-oh-TOK-sin] formation of excess bone tissue on the surface of a bone; also called an osteoma

**exotropia** [eks-oh-TROH-pee-ah] outward turning of the eyeball

**expectorate** [ek-SPEK-tor-ate] to cough up and expel mucus from the airway

**expiratory reserve volume (ERV)** [eks-PY-rah-tor-ee ree-ZEERV VOL-yoom] the volume of air exiting the lungs combined with tidal volume (TV) during forced exhalation; average value = 1,000 cc

**exploratory laparotomy** [eks-PLOR-ah-tor-ee LAP-ah-ROT-oh-mee] surgical procedure that uses an abdominal incision to open the abdominopelvic cavity for scrutiny

**exstrophy** [EK-stroh-fee] extrusion of a hollow organ, such as the bladder, causing it to be turned inside out due to congenital malformation

**extensor muscles** [eks-TEN-sur MUS-selz] muscles that extend or stretch a limb or part

**extensor muscles of the hand** [eks-TEN-sur MUS-selz uv the hand] collective group of muscles on the dorsal surface of the forearm that function to extend the hand and wrist; includes the extensor carpi, radialis longus, and radialis brevis muscles

**external** [eks-TER-nal] outside or exterior of the body or organ

**external acoustic meatus** [eks-TER-nal ah-KYOOS-tik mee-AY-tus] outer segment of the ear canal

**external carotid artery** [eks-TER-nal ka-ROT-id AR-ter-ee] a large blood vessel of the neck that carries oxygenated blood to the thyroid gland, face, throat, and mandible

**external fixation** [eks-TER-nal fik-SAY-shun] surgical procedure used to treat a complicated fracture using application of metal pins that are inserted in the bone on either side of the fracture and connected to a metal frame to immobilize a fracture or lengthen a congenitally short leg

**external genitalia** [eks-TER-nal jen-ih-TAL-ee-ah] genitalia on the outside of the body; includes the scrotum, testes, epididymis, and penis in males; and labia, clitoris, and urethra in females

**external iliac artery** [eks-TER-nal IL-ee-ak AR-ter-ee] the large, more superficial division of the common iliac artery that extends down into the thigh and becomes the femoral artery

**external jugular vein** [eks-TER-nal JUG-yoo-lar vayn] the paired, bilateral blood vessels of the neck that return blood from the head and neck to the heart

**external oblique muscle** [eks-TER-nal OH-bleek MUS-sel] a bilateral muscle of the lateral chest that begins at the fifth ribs and inserts into the anterior iliac crest, serving the function of compressing the abdomen and maintaining an upright posture

**extracellular fluid** [EKS-trah-SEL-yoo-lar FLOO-id] liquid in the body that is outside the cells

**extracorporeal** [eks-trah-kor-POR-ee-al] outside the body

**extracorporeal circulation** [eks-trah-kor-POR-ee-al sir-kyoo-LAY-shun] shunting of blood outside the body to a device that performs a body function; blood is then returned to the patient's circulatory system; examples include the use of a heart-lung machine or kidney dialysis

**extracorporeal lithotripsy** [eks-trah-kor-POR-ee-al lith-oh-TRIP-see] a therapeutic procedure in which shock waves are transmitted to the kidneys to break apart renal calculi; also known as extracorporeal shock wave lithotripsy

**extraocular** [eks-trah-OK-yoo-lar] anatomical region immediately adjacent to or near the outside surface of the eye

**extraocular muscles** [eks-trah-OK-yoo-lar MUS-selz] muscles that control the movements of the eye

**extrapyramidal side effects (EPS)** [ECKS-trah-pih-RAM-ih-dal SIDE ee-FEKTS] an untoward effect of neuroleptic medications with distressing symptoms including tremors, bradykinesia, dystonia, and restless movements of the mouth, legs, and hands

**extraurethral incontinence** [EKS-trah-yoo-re-thral in-KON-tin-ens] loss of control of urine flow caused when the sphincter mechanism has been bypassed

**extravasation** [EKS-trav-ah-SAY-shun] damage to tissue of the vein and surrounding structures when a chemotherapeutic drug leaks into the soft tissue surrounding the infusion site

**extremity** [eks-TREM-ih-tee] referring to legs, arms, and phalanges

**extrinsic asthma** [eks-TRIN-sik AZ-mah] asthma caused by an environmental allergen

**extubation** [eks-too-BAY-shun] removal of a tube, especially an endotracheal tube

**exudate** [EKS-yoo-dayt] movement of fluid from a vessel wall into a body cavity or adjacent tissue; often occurring due to inflammatory processes

**exudative** [eks-YOO-day-tiv] substance that leaks into or out of tissues

# F

**factitious disorder** [fak-TISH-us dis-OR-der] physical and/or psychological symptoms that are consciously fabricated by the patient; pretending to be sick (often with symptoms that are difficult to evaluate)

**false ribs** [FAHLS ribz] the five lower costal bones on either side of the chest that do not attach directly to the sternum

**false vocal cords** [FAHLS VOH-kal kordz] vestibular folds in the larynx that do not produce sounds

**Farre's tubercles** [FARZ TOO-ber-kulz] malignant masses on the surface of the liver

**fascia** [FASH-uh] fibrous connective tissue that covers, supports, and separate muscles

**fasciculation** [fah-sik-yoo-LAY-shun] uncontrollable, localized contraction of a single muscle group that is visible through the skin

**fasciectomy** [fash-ee-EK-toh-mee] excision of the fascia that covers the surface of a muscle

**fasciorrhaphy** [fash-ee-OR-ah-fee] suturing of the fascia that covers the surface of a muscle

**febrile** [FEE-brile] having an elevated temperature

**fecal incontinence** [FEE-kul in-KONT-in-ens] inability to control defecation

**fecalith** [FEE-kah-lith] hardened feces that become a stonelike mass, occurring most often in the appendix or a diverticulum

**feces** [FEE-seez] end product of digestion comprised of undigested fibers and liquid; also called stool

**femoral artery** [FEM-or-al AR-tur-ee] blood vessel of the medial aspect of the thigh that carries oxygenated blood; originates at the external iliac artery and terminates at the popliteal artery behind the knee

**femoral vein** [FEM-or-al vayn] blood vessel of the thigh that returns blood from the lower leg, starting at the popliteal vein and ending at the iliac vein

**femoris anterior muscle** [FEM-or-is an-TEER-ee-or MUS-sel] large muscle mass of the upper leg composed of four smaller muscles (rectus femoris, vastus lateralis, vastus medialis, and vastus intermedius), which work together to extend the leg and are often referred to simply as quadriceps

**femur** [FEE-mur] thighbone extending from the hip to the knee

**fenestra** [fe-NES-trah] small opening to relieve pressure; microscopic openings in capillaries for the purpose of filtration within the glomerular capillaries of the kidneys

**ferritin** [FAIR-ih-tin] blood chemistry test, used to diagnose iron deficiency anemia, that indirectly measures the amount of iron stored in the body by measuring the small amount that is always present in the blood

**ferrotherapy** [fer-oh-THER-ah-pee] treatment of anemia by administration of iron compounds

**fertilization** [fer-tih-ly-ZAY-shun] union of a sperm and egg that develops into an embryo

**festination** [FES-tih-nay-shun] to increase in speed or rate; commonly associated with the gait pattern of individuals with Parkinson's disease

**fetal alcohol syndrome** [FE-tal AL-ko-hol SIN-drom] fetal development which is impaired by maternal consumption of alcohol; commonly demonstrated in the infant by craniofacial abnormalities, limb defects, and some mental retardation

**fetometry** [fee-TOM-eh-tree] estimation of the size, age, and growth of a fetus using ultrasonography

**fetoscope** [FEE-toe-skope] a fibro-optical device used for direct visualization of an embryo; historical term for stethoscope used to listen to fetal heart sounds

**fibrillation** [fib-ril-LAY-shun] exceedingly rapid contractions or twitching of muscular fibrils, but not of the muscle as a whole

**fibroadenoma** [fye-bro-ad-eh-NOH-mah] formation of firm, densely fibrous, benign tumors in glandular tissue; frequently observed in the breast

**fibromyalgia** [fye-bro-migh-AL-jee-uh] widespread muscle and joint pain of unknown origin

**fibromyositis** [FYE-bro-mi-oh-SIGH-tis] chronic muscle inflammation with hyperplasia of the connective tissue

**fibroplasia** [FYE-bro-PLAY-zee-ah] overproduction of fibrous tissue

**fibrosis** [fye-BROH-sis] increase or abnormal growth of fibrous or connective tissue in reparative or reactive processes

**fibula** [FIB-yoo-lah] the anterior bone of the lower leg that extends from the knee and terminates at the lateral aspect of the ankle

**-fida** [fy-dah] *suffix*; split

**fifth cranial nerve (CN V)** [fifth KRA-nee-ahl nerv] trigeminal nerve which stimulates the face and upper neck

**filiform papillae** [FIL-ih-form pa-PIL-ee] condition of having numerous elongated cone-shaped keratinic projections on the dorsal surface of the tongue

**filtration** [fil-TRAY-shun] to strain or separate by passing liquid through a device to separate wanted from unwanted substances, as in dialysis

**fimbria** [FIM-bree-uh] finger- or fringe-shaped projections extending from the distal ends of the fallopian tubes

**first-degree burn** [FURST-de-GREE burn] damage to the epidermal layer; burned-tissue reaction as a result of thermal, radioactive, chemical, or electrical insult

**fiss-** [fis] *prefix*; a split or cleft

**fissures** [FISH-urz] cracks in the skin or other tissues

**fistula** [FIST-yoo-lah] abnormal passage that connects two structures

**flaccid** [FLAS-sid] having poor or absent muscle tone

**flaccid paralysis** [FLAS-sid par-RAHL-ih-sis] defective, poor, or absent muscle control caused by a nerve lesion

**flagellum** [fla-JEL-um] a whiplike structure that propels sperm

**flail chest** [FLAYL chest] condition where three or more consecutive ribs have fractured in close proximity; this creates instability of the wall of the thorax, moving opposite to the normal direction during respiratory movements

**flatulence** [FLAT-yoo-lens] excessive gas in the intestinal tract, in the stomach or intestines

**flatus** [FLAY-tus] intestinal gas that is the end product of bacteria in the large intestine feeding on undigested food

**flex-** [fleks] *prefix*; bend

**flexion** [FLECK-shun] bending movement at a joint

**flexor muscles** [FLEKS-or MUS-selz] muscles that bend or flex a limb or part

**floaters** [FLO-terz] clumps of gel or cellular debris within the vitreous; these are experienced as small specks seen moving across the visual field

**floating ribs** [FLO-ting ribz] the 11th and 12th ribs, which do not attach to the sternum

**fluorescein angiography** [floo-oh-RES-sen an-jee-OG-rah-fee] diagnostic procedure in which fluorescein, an orange fluorescent dye, is injected intravenously, traveling to the retinal artery in the eye and causing it to glow fluorescent green on flash photography of the retina

**fluoroscopy** [floor-OS-koh-pee] examination of deep tissues and structures of the body by x-ray using a fluoroscope

**-flux** [flux] *suffix*; flow

**focus charting** [FO-kus CHAR-ting] documentation method using a columnar format to chart data, action, and response

**Foley catheter** [FOH-lee KATH-eh-ter] a urethrally inserted urine drainage tube with an inflatable retaining balloon

**follicle** [FOL-ih-kul] space containing the hair root

**folliculitis** [fol-IK-yoo-LYE-tis] inflammation of the hair follicles

**fontanel** [fawn-tah-NEL] non-ossified membrane covering the anterior portion of the skull of a fetus; located between the cranial bones, commonly called "the soft spot"

**foramen** [foh-RAY-men] an opening in a bone through which nerves, blood vessels, and other structures pass

**foramen magnum** [foh-RAY-men MAG-num] a large opening at the base of the cranium near the occipital bone that the spinal cord passes through as it connects with the medulla oblongata

**forebrain** [FOR-brayn] the anterior portion of the brain including the telencephalon and diencephalon

**-form** [form] *suffix*; having the manner or structure of

**formication** [for-mih-KAY-shun] tactile hallucination or sensation that small insects are crawling under the skin; frequently associated with alcohol detoxification

**fornix** [FOR-niks] a tract of myelinated nerves along the arched floor of the lateral ventricles, connecting the hippocampus in each temporal lobe to the thalamus and each amygdaloid body

**fossa** [FAW-sah] a shallow depression in a bone or tissue

**fourth cranial nerve (CN IV)** [forth KRA-nee-ahl nerv] trochlear nerve; innervates the sensory and motor function of the superior oblique muscle of the eye

**fourth heart sound** [forth hart sownd] sound produced by the heart during late systole due to ventricular atrial systole and decreased ventricular compliances; often associated with ventricular hypertrophy, hypertension, and myocardial infarction

**fovea** [FOH-vee-ah] a natural depression on a body surface such as a bone

**fovea visuala** [FOH-vee-ah viz-OO-ah-lah] a small depression in the center of the macula, directly opposite the pupil, where the greatest visual acuity lies

**Fowler position** [FOW-ler po-ZISH-un] semireclining in bed, with head of bed elevated

**fracture** [FRAK-chur] breakage of bone due to injury or disease process; classified according to the direction of the break or degree of disruption of structural integrity

**fragile X syndrome** [FRAJ-il ex SIN-drom] a disorder caused by extra genetic fragments on the X chromosome, resulting in mental retardation, distinctive facial deformity, and macro-orchidism

**free radicals** [free RAD-ih-kalz] atoms or groups of atoms that can cause damage to cells

**fremitus** [FREM-ih-tus] palpable vibration; crackles or thrill from body cavities or joints; subtypes include tactile, vocal, and tussive

**frenulum** [FREN-yoo-lum] an elongated connective structure that attaches two parts such as the posterior surface of the tongue and upper lip at the gum line

**friction rub** [FRIK-shun rub] abnormal grating sounds detected during auscultation when pleura or pericardial tissues are inflamed

**frontal bone** [FRON-tal bohn] large bone of the cranium that forms the forehead and superior portions of the orbits

**frontal lobe** [FRON-tal lohb] the portion of each cerebral hemisphere located anterior to the central sulcus

**frontal sinus** [FRON-tal SY-nus] a hollow space in the area of the forehead

**frontalis muscle** [fron-TAL-is MUS-sel] muscle that covers the frontal bone

**fructosuria** [FRUK-tos-YUR-ee-ah] excretion of fructose in the urine

**-fuge** [fyooj] *suffix*; to drive away; having a fleeting quality

**fulguration** [ful-gyoo-RAY-shun] destruction of unwanted tissue by the use of electrical current in the form of sparks

**full thickness graft** [ful THIK-nes graft] surgical transplantation of the epidermis and underlying tissues

**fundus** [FUN-dus] the area furthest from the opening

**fungating** [FUN-gayt-ing] rapid growth similar to fungus; used to describe some quick-developing tumors

**furuncle** [FUR-ung-kul] a boil

**fusiform aneurysm** [FEW-zi-form AN-yoo-riz-um] spindle-shaped protrusion on an artery

# G

**gag reflex** [GAG REE-fleks] response by the throat that causes retching

**gait apraxia** [gayt ah-PRAK-see-uh] loss of the ability to consciously sequence and execute the movements required to coordinate walking, resulting in unsteady walking patterns; widely based, jerky gait, and balance difficulties as demonstrated in Parkinson's disease

**galactocele** [ga-LAK-tow-seel] a cyst caused by an occluded lactiferous duct in the breast

**gallbladder** [GALL-blad-der] a pear-shaped pouch on the inferior surface of the right hepatic lobe that stores bile

**gallium** [GAL-ee-um] a radioisotope utilized in diagnostic scans for neoplasm, inflammation, and soft-tissue disorders

**gamete** [GAM-eet] spermatozoa from the male or ova from the female; cells that have only 23 chromosomes rather than the usual 46

**gamma-amino butyric acid (GABA)** [GAM-ah-ah-MEE-noh byu-TER-ik AS-id] an amino acid that functions as an inhibitory neurotransmitter in the brain and spinal cord

**ganglion cyst** [GANG-lee-on sist] a fluid-filled mass most often observed in the wrist, but may also occur on the ankle

**ganglionectomy** [gang-glee-ohn-EK-tuh-mee] excision of a ganglion

**ganglionic cyst** [GANG-glee-ohn-ik sist] a benign cyst localized on or around a tendon sheath or joint capsule

**gangrene** [GANG-green] necrosis of a body tissue

**gastralgia** [gas-TRAL-gee-uh] pain in the stomach

**gastrectomy** [gas-TREK-toh-mee] surgical removal of part or all of the stomach

**gastric** [GAS-trik] pertaining to the stomach

**gastric bypass** [GAS-trik BY-pass] surgical creation of a small stomach pouch with anastomosis of the stomach with the jejunum, reducing caloric absorption as a treatment for morbid obesity

**gastrinoma** [gas-trin-OH-mah] a tumor associated with Zollinger-Ellison syndrome that secretes gastrin

**gastritis** [gas-TRY-tis] acute or chronic inflammation of the stomach due to excess acid production or a bacterial infection

**gastrocele** [GAS-troh-seel] herniation or protrusion of part of the stomach

**gastrocnemius muscle** [gas-trok-NEE-mee-us MUS-sel] muscle of the posterior surface of the lower leg that, when flexed, initiates plantar flexion

**gastroenteritis** [gas-troh-en-tur-EYE-tis] stomach and intestinal inflammation resulting from infection

**gastroenterologist** [gas-troh-en-ter-AWL-oh-jist] physician who practices in the medical specialty of gastroenterology, diagnosing and treating patients with diseases of the gastrointestinal system

**gastroenterology** [gas-troh-EN-ter-AWL-oh-jee] study of the stomach and intestines

**gastroesophageal** [gas-troh-ee-sof-ah-JEE-ul] pertaining to the esophagus and stomach

**gastroesophageal reflux disease** [gas-troh-ee-sof-ah-JEE-ul REE-fluks dis-EEZ] disorder of stomach contents being regurgitated into the esophagus

**gastrointestinal** [gas-troh-en-TES-tih-nal] pertaining to the stomach and intestines

**gastroparesis** [gas-troh-pah-REE-sis] reduced contractility of the stomach

**gastroplasty** [GAS-troh-plas-tee] surgical procedure for severe obesity in which the size and volume capacity of the stomach are reduced by staples or intestinal bypass

**gastrorrhaphy** [gas-TROR-ah-fee] suturing or sewing an injured stomach wall

**gastroscopy** [GAS-tros-skop-ee] visualization of the esophagus, stomach, and duodenum using a fiberoptic endoscope

**gastrospasm** [GAS-troh-spazm] sudden, involuntary, and painful contraction of the stomach muscles

**gastrostomy** [gas-TROWS-toh-mee] surgical creation of a permanent opening from the abdominal wall into the stomach to insert a gastrostomy tube

**-gen** [jen] *suffix*; production or origin

**-genesis** [jen-ee-sis] *suffix*; produce or originate

**genital** [JEN-ih-tal] pertaining to the reproductive organs of male and female

**genitourinary system** [JEN-ih-toh-YOO-rih-nair-ee SIS-tem] comprised of the kidney, ureters, and bladder

**genotype** [JEN-oh-type] the genetic makeup of an individual

**genu valgum** [JEEN-yoo VAL-gum] congenital deformity in which the lower legs are bent medially; also known as knock-knee

**genu varum** [JEEN-yoo VA-rum] congenital deformity in which the lower legs are bent away from the midline; also known as bowleg

**geriatrics** [jer-ee-AT-riks] branch of medicine dealing with care and treatment of problems particular to old age

**germinal cell** [JER-min-al sell] a tissue from which other tissues or cells proliferate

**germinal centers** [JER-min-al SEN-terz] areas of rapidly dividing lymphocytes within the lymph nodules that respond to infection by forming and releasing lymphocytes for combat

**germinal stage** [JER-min-al STAYJ] developmental stage that begins with conception and lasts approximately 10 to 14 days

**gero-** [jer-oh] *prefix*; elderly, old age

**gerontology** [jer-on-TOL-oh-jee] the study of the problems particular to old age and the aging process

**gestalt therapy** [ges-TALT THAIR-ah-pee] a form of psychotherapy that emphasizes treating the whole person by focusing on relationships and responses both emotional and biological

**gestation** [jes-TAY-shun] length of time of the development of a fetus in utero from conception to birth

**gestational diabetes mellitus** [jes-TAY-shun-al dye-ah-BEE-teez mel-EYE-tus] disorder of glucose metabolism that occurs during pregnancy; type III

**giardiasis** [jee-ar-DI-aye-sis] infection with the parasite *Giardia lamblia* which causes diarrhea, cramping, and dyspepsia

**gingival hyperplasia** [jin-JYH-val hy-per-PLAY-zee-uh] overgrowth of gum tissue commonly observed in patients treated with anticonvulsants

**gingivitis** [jin-jih-VY-tis] inflammation of the tissue (gums) immediately adjacent to the teeth

**gingivoglossitis** [JIN-jih-voh-glaw-SY-tis] inflammation of the gums and tongue

**gland** [gland] any one of many organs in the body comprised of specialized cells that secrete or excrete materials not related to their ordinary metabolism

**Glasgow coma scale** [GLAS-goh KOH-mah SKAYL] a clinical observation scale used to document level of consciousness

**glaucoma** [glaw-KOH-mah] increased intraocular pressure (IOP) because the aqueous humor cannot circulate freely; in open-angle glaucoma, the angle where the edges of the iris and cornea touch is normal and open, but the trabecular meshwork is blocked

**glenoid** [GLEH-noyd] resembling a socket of a joint; the depressed or indented articular surface

**glenoid cavity** [GLEH-noyd KAV-ih-tee] the depression in the scapula into which the head of the humerus fits

**glenoid fossa** [GLEH-noyd FAW-sah] a shallow depression where the head of the humerus joins the scapula to make the shoulder joint

**-glia** [glee-ah] *suffix*; substance that holds matter together

**glioma** [GLEE-oh-mah] tumor of glial cells graded by degree of invasion

**global amnesia** [GLOH-bal am-NEE-zee-ah] loss of all memories

**glomerular filtration** [gloh-MER-yoo-lur fil-TRAY-shun] the rate at which blood is filtered at the glomerulus; clearance test used to determine the glomerular filtrating rate

**glomerulonephritis** [gloh-mer-yoo-loh-nef-RIGH-tis] an inflammatory disease of the kidney typically occurring one to two weeks after a streptococcal bacterial infection; symptoms include hematuria and proteinuria

**glomerulosclerosis** [gloh-mer-yoo-loh-skle-ROH-sis] fibrosis of the renal glomeruli

**glossal** [GLOS-al] relating to the tongue

**glossectomy** [glaw-SEK-toh-mee] surgical revision or complete excision of the tongue

**glossitis** [glaw-SY-tis] inflammation of the tongue which may be caused by irritation from food, infection, or vitamin B deficiency

**glottis** [GLOT-tis] the vocal apparatus of the larynx, including the vocal folds, vocal chords, vocal muscles, and adjacent structures of the throat

**glucagon** [GLOO-kuh-gon] pancreatic hormone from alpha cells that elevates blood glucose

**glucogenesis** [glu-koh-JEN-eh-sis] formation of sugar from fats and proteins

**glucometer** [GLU-koh-mee-ter] a device used to measure blood levels of glucose

**glucose tolerance test** [GLU-kos TOL-er-ans test] diagnostic study in which the patient is administered 75 g of glucose while fasting, with measurement of blood glucose at regular intervals to determine ability to regulate glucose metabolism

**glucosuria** [GLOO-kohs-YOOR-ee-ah] presence of glucose (sugar) in the urine

**gluten enteropathy** [GLOO-tin en-tur-OWP-ah-thee] malabsorption and gastric irritation due to gluten sensitivity; celiac sprue, celiac disease

**gluteus** [GLYOO-tee-us] referring to the buttocks

**gluteus maximus muscle** [GLYOO-tee-us MAK-sih-mus MUS-sel] large muscle forming the buttocks that extends to the thigh

**gluteus medius muscle** [GLYOO-tee-us MEE-dee-us MUS-sel] middle, smaller muscle in the buttock region that extends to the thigh

**glycohemoglobin** [GLYE-ko-HEE-moh-glo-bin] a hemoglobin A molecule with a glucose group on the N-terminal valine amino acid unit of the beta chain

**glycolysis** [gly-KOL-ih-sis] energy-yielding conversion of glucose to lactic acid in the tissues

**glycosylated hemoglobin** [GLYE-kos-ih-lay-ted HEE-moh-gloh-ben] used to test circulating glucose blood levels over the life span of a red blood cell

**gnath-** [nath] *prefix*; pertaining to the jaw and/or cheek

**gnathoplasty** [NATH-oh-plas-tee] surgical reconstruction of the jaw

**-gogue** [gog] *suffix*; to make flow

**goiter** [GOY-tur] enlargement of the thyroid gland

**goniometer** [goh-nee-AWM-eh-ter] a protractor-like device used to measure the angle and degrees of range of movement (ROM) of a joint

**gonioscopy** [goh-nee-AWS-koh-pee] use of a slit lamp with a special lens that illuminates the trabecular meshwork

**gonococcus** [gon-oh-KOK-us] infectious agent in the sexually transmitted disease gonorrhea

**gonorrhea** [gon-oh-REE-ah] a sexually transmitted disease caused by the microorganism *Neisseria gonorrhea* causing inflammation of the urethra, endocervix, and fallopian tubes

**gout** [GOWT] disorder that occurs most often in men due to excessive levels of uric acid in the blood; acute attacks cause sudden, severe pain in the great toe or hands as uric acid moves from the blood into the soft tissues and forms masses of crystals with soft-tissue swellings known as tophi

**gouty arthritis** [GOW-tee arth-RY-tis] inflammation of joints due to formation of tophi from accumulation of uric acid crystals

**gracilis muscle** [GRAS-ih-lis MUS-sel] skeletal muscle that inserts near the pubis and extends to the medial tuberosity of the tibia; upon contraction it adducts the thigh and flexes the knee

**graft** [GRAFT] surgical procedure that uses skin, whole bone, or bone chips to repair areas of tissue damage

**-gram** [gram] *suffix*; record of

**-graph** [graf] *suffix;* instrument that records

**-graphy** [graf-ee] *suffix;* process of recording data

**Graves disease** [GRAYVZ dis-EEZ] a form of hyperthyroidism caused by excessive thyroid hormone production, resulting in enlargement of the thyroid gland and exophthalmos

**-gravida** [grav-id-ah] *suffix;* pregnancy

**gray matter** [gray MAT-er] brain and spinal-cord tissue made up primarily of unmyelinated fibers of cell bodies and dendrites of nerve cells

**great saphenous vein** [grayt sah-FEE-nus vayn] major blood vessel that returns blood along the medial surface of the thigh

**greenstick fracture** [GREEN-stik FRAK-shur] a break in bone with disruption of structure only on one side; occurs most often in children, as part of the bone is still composed of flexible cartilage

**gross** [GROHS] visible to the naked eye; large in size

**guaiac** [GWY-ak] a solution used to test for the presence of occult blood in fecal matter

**gustation** [gus-TAY-shun] sense of taste

**Guthrie's test** [GUTH-reez test] a routine screening test for phenylketonuria in newborns consisting of placing a small amount of blood on filter paper to detect the presence of excessive phenylalanine in the blood

**gynecologist** [gye-neh-KOL-oh-jist] a physician specializing in the study of diseases and treatment of the female genital tract

**gynecomastia** [GY-neh-koh-MAS-tee-ah] development of excessive mammary ducts or tissues in males due to mildly increased estrogen levels

**-gynous** [gin-us] *suffix;* having female characteristics

**gyrus** [JY-rus] a bulge or convolution on the surface of the cerebral cortex of the brain

# H

**H2 receptor antagonist** [aitch-too ree-SEP-tor an-TAG-oh-nist] drug that blocks gastric secretions; proton or pump inhibition for the purpose of suppressing gastric acid secretion

**hair cells** [HAIR SELZ] epithelial cells with hairlike processes that respond to sound waves and maintain equilibrium

**hair follicle** [HAIR FOL-ih-kel] a saclike structure from which hair grows

**hairline fracture** [HAIR-lyne FRAK-shur] a very thin break line of the bone with pieces closely approximated, which is often difficult to detect on an x-ray

**half-life** [HAF-lyf] time required by the body to eliminate half of the blood concentration level of the original drug dose

**Hallervorden-Spatz syndrome** [HOL-eh-FOR-den-shpots SIN-drom] a degenerative neurological disorder found in children; characterized by parkinsonism, rigidity, and progressive dementia due to accumulation of iron pigments in the brain

**hallucination** [hal-loo-sih-NAY-shun] subjective perception of events and sensations for which there is no external basis

**hallucinatory neuralgia** [ha-LOO-sen-ah-tor-ee nyoo-RAL-jee-ah] sensation of localized pain following the cessation of an episode of severe throbbing pain

**hallucinogen** [huh-LOO-sih-noh-jen] a drug such as LSD or PCP that reduces perceptions of reality

**hallucis flexus** [HAL-yoo-sis FLEK-sus] permanent contracture of the great toe; commonly referred to as a hammertoe

**hallux** [HAL-uks] great toe, which is on the medial side of the foot

**hallux rigidus** [HAL-uks rih-JID-us] a painful condition of the great toe where the joint cartilage deteriorates at the articular surface of the metatarsal, resulting in painful ambulation and stiffening of the joint

**hallux valgus** [HAL-uks VAL-gus] deformity of the foot in which the great toe is angled laterally toward the other toes

**halo traction** [HAY-loh TRAK-shun] use of pins inserted into the cranium and attached to a circular metal ring, forming a halo and stabilizing cervical fractures

**hamate** [HAM-ayt] one of eight carpal bones located on the distal portion of the wrist

**hamstring muscle group** [HAM-string MUS-sel GRUP] a collective mass of muscles of the upper posterior leg that flex the leg; composed of biceps femoris, semitendinosus, and semimembranosus muscles

**hard palate** [hard PAL-ayte] the anterior bony portion of the roof of the mouth that contains the palatine vessels, nerves, and mucous glands

**Hashimoto's thyroiditis** [hah-shee-MOH-tohz THIGH-roid-eye-tis] autoimmune disease causing an inflamed thyroid gland

**haustra** [HOS-tra] pouchlike structures in the intestinal walls that expand and contract to hold varying amounts of food during digestion

**Haversian canals** [ha-VER-zhan kah-NALZ] nutrient system within compact bone that contains nerves, blood vessels, and lymphatic vessels

**heart** [HART] the hollow muscular organ responsible for acting as a pump for the circulation of blood

**heart failure** [hart FAIL-yer] condition in which the heart cannot pump enough blood to meet the metabolic requirement of body tissues due to myocardial infarction, ischemic heart disease, or cardiomyopathy

**heart-lung machine** [hart-LUNG mah-SHEEN] mechanical device that serves as artificial lungs and heart during some cardiac procedures

**hebephrenia** [HEB-ee-FREE-nee-ah] a trait associated with schizophrenia in which the patient demonstrates childish or silly behavior

**Heimlich maneuver** [HYM-lik man-OOV-er] procedure used to assist individuals with airway obstruction due to choking by grasping around the victim's waist from behind and applying a forceful push upward and inward to generate a burst of air to remove the obstruction

*Helicobacter pylori* [hel-ih-koh-BAK-ter py-LOR-eye] bacterium thought to be responsible for the majority of gastric ulcer diseases

**hem-** [heem] *prefix*; blood

**hemangioma** [hee-MAN-jee-OH-ma] congenital proliferation of blood vessels resulting in a mass; occurs frequently in the skin and subcutaneous tissue

**hemarthrosis** [HEE-mar-THROH-sis] blood in the joint cavity from blunt trauma or penetrating wound, or occurring spontaneously in hemophiliac patients

**hematemesis** [hem-ah-TEM-esis] vomiting of new or old blood from bleeding stomach or esophagus; can be caused by an esophageal ulcer, esophageal varix, or gastric ulcer

**hematochezia** [he-MAH-toh-KEE-zee-ah] blood in the stool due to an ulcer, Crohn's disease, polyp, diverticulum, or hemorrhoid

**hematocrit** [hee-MAT-oh-krit] a laboratory test that determines the percentage of erythrocytes in a blood sample

**hematologist** [HEE-mah-TAWL-oh-jist] physician who practices the medical specialty of blood disorders and blood-forming tissues

**hematometra** [HEE-mah-toh-ME-trah] collection of blood in the uterine cavity

**hematuria** [hee-muh-TUR-ee-ah] abnormal presence of blood in the urine

**hemi-** [hem-ee] *prefix*; one-half

**hemianalgesia** [HEM-ee-an-al-JEE-zee-ah] loss of sensitivity to pain on one side of the body

**hemianopia** [HEM-ee-ah-NOH-pee-ah] loss of vision in half of the normal visual field (right or left, top or bottom)

**hemiataxia** [HEM-ee-ah-TAX-ee-ah] loss of muscular control affecting one side of the body, often due to stroke or traumatic injury of the cerebellum

**hemiazygos vein** [HEM-ee-ah-ZY-gos vayn] one of the blood vessels of the thorax that begins in the left ascending lumbar vein, proceeds through the thorax, and eventually goes up to the azygous vein

**hemicolectomy** [HEM-ih-koh-LEK-toh-mee] excision of half of the colon

**hemiparesis** [HEM-ee-pah-REE-sis] partial paralysis; weakness on the right or left half of the body

**hemiplegia** [hem-ee-PLE-jee-ah] paralysis on one side of the body

**hemiplegic gait** [hem-ee-PLE-jik gayt] manner of walking with a stiff, extended leg, lacking any flexion of the knee or ankle, resulting in a semicircular movement of the foot with each step

**hemispasm** [HEM-ee-spazm] involuntary, painful muscular contractions of one side of the body or face

**hemodialysis** [hem-oh-dye-AL-ih-sis] filtering of blood through an external machine that stands in for the kidneys; used in cases of renal failure and some toxic conditions

**hemodialyzer** [hem-oh-DYE-uh-lye-zur] machine that acts as an artificial kidney during dialysis

**hemodynamics** [HEE-moh-dy-NAM-iks] pressures generated by blood and passage of blood through the heart and pulmonary system

**hemoglobin A** [HEE-moh-gloh-bin AYE] normal hemoglobin that binds with oxygen and carbon dioxide

**hemolytic uremic syndrome** [hem-oh-LIT-ik ur-REE-mik SIN-drom] a rare kidney disorder with onset usually in infancy that presents with renal failure, destruction of red blood cells, and platelet deficiency; treatment includes dialysis and conservative treatment with good prognosis for infants and children, but less optimistic outcomes for adults

**hemophilia** [HEE-moh-FIL-ee-ah] an inherited genetic abnormality of a gene on the X chromosome, causing a lack or a deficiency of a specific clotting factor; disorder causes permanent tendency toward spontaneous and traumatic episodes of hemorrhage

**hemophilia A** [HEE-moh-FIL-ee-ah AYE] inherited blood disorder resulting in the absence of clotting factor VIII; this is the most common type of hemophilia, occurring almost exclusively in males

**hemophilia B** [HEE-moh-FIL-ee-ah BEE] inherited blood disorder resulting in the absence of clotting factor IX

**hemophilia C** [HEE-moh-FIL-ee-ah SEE] inherited blood disorder resulting in the absence of clotting factor XI

**hemoptysis** [hee-MOP-ti-sis] coughing up blood or blood-tinged mucus

**hemorrhagic stroke** [hem-oh-RAJ-ik STROK] sudden bleeding in the brain that disrupts the supply of nutrients to the brain

**hemorrhoid** [HEM-or-royd] swollen, protruding veins in the rectum; usually described as being internal or external

**hemosiderosis** [HEE-moh-sid-er-OH-sis] increased storage of iron in body tissues; associated with diseases involving the destruction of red blood cells; for example, hemolytic anemia

**hemostasis** [HEE-moh-stay-sis] to stop bleeding; stabilize input and output of a system

**hemostatic forceps** [hee-moh-STAT-ik FORE-seps] clamping tool with a clasp that holds the blades in a closed position; used to stop blood flow at the end of a blood vessel and control hemorrhage; often called "hemostat"

**hemothorax** [hem-oh-THOR-aks] abnormal presence of blood in the pleural cavity

**hepatatoiminodiacetic scan (HIDA)** [HEP-ah-tah-toh-IM-in-oh-dy-ah-SEE-tik skan] a diagnostic imaging technique of injection of the radionuclide to obtain images of the liver, gallbladder, and biliary tree

**hepatic portal** [he-PAT-ik POR-tul] the pathway of blood flow from the gastrointestinal (GI) tract and spleen to the liver via the portal vein and its tributaries

**hepatic portal circulation** [he-PAT-ik POR-tul sir-kyoo-LAY-shun] blood vessels that divert blood from digestive organs to the liver before returning through veins back up to the heart

**hepatic portal vein** [he-PAT-ik POR-tul vayn] blood vessel that carries blood from the liver to the inferior vena cava

**hepatitis A** [hep-ah-TY-tis aye] inflammation of the liver due to infection from hepatitis A virus that is most often transmitted through contact with contaminated food or water; may be transmitted between sexual partners

**hepatitis B** [hep-ah-TY-tis bee] inflammation of the liver due to infection with the hepatitis B virus; symptoms may be acute or chronic, and include jaundice, nausea, vomiting, and joint pain; infection may be transmitted between sexual partners and by blood-borne exposure

**hepatitis C** [hep-ah-TY-tis see] inflammation of the liver due to infection with a single-stranded RNA virus by way of blood or body fluids; typical presentation of persistent elevation of liver enzymes on routine lab testing; may be transmitted between sexual partners

**hepatocyte** [hep-AH-toh-site] cell of liver tissue

**hepatoma** [hep-ah-TOH-ma] neoplastic or benign tumors of the liver

**hepatomegaly** [HEP-ah-toh-MEG-ah-lee] palpable abdominal enlargement of the liver due to damage from cirrhosis or hepatitis

**hepatosplenomegaly** [HEP-ah-toh-sple-noh-MEG-ah-lee] enlargement of both the liver and the spleen

**hepatotoxic** [HEP-ah-toh-TOK-sik] having an overwhelmingly detrimental or destructive effect on the liver; for example, large doses of acetaminofen

**hereditary disease** [heh-RED-ih-tair-ee dis-EEZ] illness caused by inherited or spontaneously mutated genetic material of the cell

**hernia** [HUR-nee-ah] abnormal protrusion of an organ through a wall or cavity

**hernia, inguinal** [HUR-nee-ah, ING-gwih-nal] protrusion of abdominal structures or bowel in the groin region

**hernia, reducible** [HUR-nee-ah, re-DEW-si-bul] abnormal protrusion of an organ through a wall or cavity that can be physically manipulated back into normal position

**herniated disc** [HER-nee-ay-ted disk] protrusion of a degenerated or fragmented intervertebral disc which often causes compression of the nerve root

**herniorrhaphy** [her-nee-OR-ah-fee] surgical repair of an opening in the wall of a body or cavity

**herpes simplex** [HER-peez SIM-pleks] recurrent, painful clusters of blisters, erupting on the lips or nose and caused by infection with herpes simplex virus type 1; after the initial infection the virus is dormant in the skin until triggers of stress, sunlight, illness, or menstruation cause it to erupt again

**herpes varicella** [HER-peez var-ih-SELL-ah] virus that causes chickenpox

**herpes zoster** [HER-peez ZOS-tur] painful raised lesions along nerve roots; also called shingles

**hertz** [HERTS] pitch or frequency of a tone is measured in hertz (Hz)

**hiatal hernia** [high-AY-tul HUR-nee-ah] protrusion of the stomach and abdominal contents through the hiatal opening due to weakness in the diaphragm

**Hickman catheter** [HIK-man KATH-eh-ter] a central venous catheter used for administration of fluids, chemotherapy, and total parental nutrition

**high-density lipoproteins** [hy-DEN-sih-tee ly-poh-PRO-teenz] a fat and protein complex that removes excess cholesterol from arterial walls and transports it to the liver

**hilar** [HY-lar] pertaining to the indented surface of the lung

**hilum** [HY-lum] an indented surface of the lung; plural is hila

**hindbrain** [HYND-brayn] the posterior area of the brain that includes the pons and cerebellum

**hippocampus** [hip-oh-KAM-pus] an elongated structure with a head and a tail that is located in each temporal lobe; responsible for controlling long-term memory and facilitating comparison between present and past emotions and experiences

**Hirschsprung's disease** [HERSH-sproongz dis-EEZ] a congenital disorder characterized by absence of autonomic parasympathetic ganglion cells in the colon that prevents peristalsis at the diverticulum causing inadequate gastric motility and mechanical obstruction of the intestine

**hirsutism** [HUR-sewt-iz-um] abnormal or excessive hair growth on a female's face or body

**His bundle** [HIZ BUN-del] a concentration of modified cardiac fibers that conduct electronic impulses to the ventricles, ultimately dividing into the left and right bundle branches

**histamine** [HIS-tah-meen] a depressor amine with powerful stimulation of gastric secretions, constriction of smooth muscle, and vasodilation

**histamine test** [HIS-tah-meen test] a diagnostic test to determine the maximal production of gastric acidity following the administration of an antihistamine subcutaneously while gastric contents are removed by a nasogastric tube for laboratory analysis

**histocyte** [HISS-toh-syt] a phagocytic cell present in connective tissue; occurs naturally as part of the body's immune system

**histology** [his-TAWL-oh-jee] study of tissues

**Hodgkin's disease** [HOJ-kins dis-EEZ] malignant lymphoma with characteristic large multinucleated cells, occurring in a single lymph node of the neck, axilla, or groin, spreading to adjacent nodes and tissues if left untreated

**Hofmeister operation** [HAWF-my-ster op-er-AYE-shun] partial gastrectomy with suturing of the lesser curvature of the stomach and anastomosis of the jejunum

**Holter monitor** [hol-ter MON-ih-ter] recording of cardiac activity by a portable device which the patient wears for as long as 24 hours

**Homans sign** [HO-manz syn] presence of pain in the calf of the leg with dorsiflexion of the foot that is indicative of thrombophlebitis or thrombosis

**homeostasis** [HOH-mee-oh-STAY-sis] condition of equilibrium in which the internal state of the body is maintained by ongoing processes of feedback and regulatory functions in response to internal and external conditions

**homicidal ideation** [HOHM-ih-SY-dal EYE-dee-AA-shun] to have thoughts, ideas, or plans to commit murder or serious bodily harm to another person as a symptom of a psychiatric disorder or delirium

**homo-** [hoh-moh] *prefix*; same or alike

**hordeolum** [hor-DEE-oh-lum] red, painful swelling or pimple containing pus near the edge of the eyelid that is caused by a bacterial infection (*Staphylococcus*) in a sebaceous (meibomian) gland

**horizontal fissure** [hor-ih-ZON-tal FISH-ur] anatomical landmark of the right lung that separates the superior and middle lobes

**horizontal plane** [hor-ih-ZON-tal PLAYN] level to the ground

**hormone** [HOR-mohn] chemical messenger found in the blood

**hormone-replacement therapy** [HOR-mohn-ree-PLAYS-ment THER-a-pee] hormone administration to restore normal function

**hospice** [HOS-pis] an end-of-life, multidisciplinary treatment provided to clients experiencing the end months of life; focuses on palliation, or relief of suffering

**human growth hormone (HGH)** [HYOO-man grohth HOR-mohn] substance secreted by the anterior pituitary gland that regulates cellular division and protein synthesis required for normal growth of tissues

**human immunodeficiency virus (HIV)** [HYOO-man im-YOO-noh-de-FISH-en-see VY-rus] retrovirus that causes acquired immunodeficiency syndrome (AIDS), resulting in loss of immune function and subsequent opportunistic infections

**human papilloma virus (HPV)** [HYOO-man pap-il-LOH-mah VY-rus] a sexually transmitted agent that causes genital warts and severe cervical intraepithelial neoplasia; it is a precursor to cervical cancer

**humerus** [HYOO-mer-us] the long bone in the upper arm that articulates with the scapula at the shoulder joint and the head of the radius and ulna to form the elbow joint

**humoral immunity** [HUGH-mor-ul im-YOO-ni-tee] immune response maintained by antibodies; antigens stimulate the production of an antibody

**Huntington's chorea** [HUN-ting-tunz koh-REE-ah] a hereditary disease of the central nervous system characterized by bizarre involuntary movements and progressive dementia

**hyaline membrane disease** [HY-ah-lin MEM-brayn dis-EEZ] respiratory disease characterized by a collapsed alveoli due to the lack of surfactant, a substance produced by the lungs to keep the alveoli inflated

**hydrarthrosis** [hy-drar-THRO-sis] accumulation of serous fluid in a joint

**hydro-** [high-droh] *prefix*; water or fluid

**hydrocele** [HY-dro-seel] any accumulation of fluid around the testicle

**hydrocephalus** [high-dro-SEF-ah-lus] abnormal accumulation of cerebrospinal fluid in the ventricles of the brain as a result of developmental anomalies, infection, or tumor

**hydrochloric acid** [HIGH-droh-klor-ik AS-id] an aqueous solution of hydrogen chloride

**hydrometer** [HIGH-droh-mee-ter] a device used to determine the specific gravity of liquid by comparison to water

**hydronephrosis** [high-droh-neh-FROH-sis] dilation of the renal pelvis and calyces of one or both kidneys due to mechanical obstruction of the flow of urine by tumor, calculus, or inflammation or obstruction of the prostate or edema

**hydrosalpinx** [hy-droh-SAL-pinks] serous fluid in the fallopian tube

**hydrosis** [high-DROH-sis] sweat production and excretion

**hydroxycorticosteroid** [high-DROK-see-kor-ti-koh-STER-oid] analysis of urine to detect cortisol byproducts

**hymen** [HY-men] thin membranous folds of tissue that partially occlude the ostium of the vagina; it is sometimes absent or disrupted even without sexual activity

**hyoid bone** [HY-oyd bohn] a flat, U-shaped bone that does not touch any other bones but functions as a bony bridge that anchors the muscles of the tongue

**hyper-** [high-per] *prefix*; above, elevated

**hyperaldosteronism** [HY-per-al-DOS-ter-ohn-izm] excessive production of aldosterone altering the regulation of potassium and sodium exchange in the distal renal tubule

**hyperalimentation** [HY-per-al-ih-men-TAY-shun] enteral or parenteral infusion of a solution containing complete nutritional requirements for normal growth, development, and tissue repair

**hyperbilirubinemia** [hy-per-BIL-ih-roo-bih-NEE-mee-uh] an abnormally high concentration of bilirubin in the circulating blood, resulting in jaundice

**hypercalcemia** [high-per-kal-SEE-mee-ah] abnormally high level of calcium in the blood

**hypercapnia** [high-per-CAP-nee-ah] abnormally high level of carbon dioxide ($CO_2$) in the arterial blood

**hyperemesis** [high-per-EM-eh-sis] extremely severe vomiting

**hyperesthesia** [HIGH-per-es-THE-zee-ah] increased sensitivity to stimulation such as pressure or touch, resulting in pain

**hyperextension** [HIGH-per-eks-TEN-shun] overstraightening; overextending beyond normal joint function or near the maximum extension

**hyperglycemia** [high-per-gly-SEE-mee-ah] abnormally high blood glucose level

**hyperinsulinism** [high-per-IN-soo-lin-izm] overproduction of insulin by the pancreas

**hyperkalemia** [high-per-ka-LEE-mee-ah] an abnormally high level of potassium in the blood

**hyperkeratosis** [HIGH-per-ker-ah-TOH-sis] overgrowth of the horny layer of the mucous membrane or epidermis

**hyperkinesis** [HIGH-per-kih-NEE-sis] excessive movement or activity; possible causes include hyperthyroidism or attention deficit disorder

**hyperlipidemia** [HIGH-per-lip-ih-DEE-mee-uh] presence of excessive amount of fats in the blood that may eventually lead to atherosclerosis

**hypermetropia** [high-per-meh-TROH-pee-uh] farsightedness; an error of refraction in which faraway objects appear more focused and clear than near objects

**hypernatremia** [high-per-nah-TREE-mee-ah] excessive level of sodium ions in the blood

**hyperopia** [HIGH-per-OH-pee-ah] farsightedness; inability to see objects in near visual fields clearly

**hyperparathyroidism** [high-per-pair-uh-THIGH-roid-izm] increased activity of parathyroid glands causing excessive parathyroid hormone (PTH) production

**hyperpnea** [high-purp-NEE-uh] increased depth and rate of respirations

**hyperresonance** [high-per-REZ-oh-nants] loud, very low-pitched, booming sounds usually heard over superinflated lungs

**hypersensitivity** [HIGH-per-sen-si-TIV-ih-tee] abnormal sensitivity to an allergen

**hypertension** [high-pur-TEN-shun] elevated blood pressure on a consistent basis with potential to cause damage to the blood vessels

**hyperthyroidism** [high-pur-THIGH-roid-iz-um] disorder of thyroid gland characterized by excessive thyroid hormone production

**hypertonic fluid** [high-per-TAWN-ik FLOO-id] liquid that is more concentrated than normal body fluid; for example, concentrated fluids used to administer some medications

**hypertrichosis** [high-pur-tri-KOH-sis] excessive growth of hair

**hypertrophy** [hy-PER-troh-fee] increase in size

**hyperuricemia** [high-pur-yoo-ri-SEE-mee-ah] elevated uric acid levels in the blood which cause nausea, anorexia, pruritus, and uremic frost

**hyperventilation** [high-pur-ven-ti-LAY-shun] increased or rapid respiratory rate that produces low alveolar carbon dioxide levels

**hyphema** [high-FEE-mah] blood in the anterior chamber of the eye, caused by trauma or increased intraocular pressure; treatment includes corticosteroid eyedrops or oral drugs

**hypo-** [high-poh] *prefix*; below, deficient or depressed

**hypoalbuminemia** [high-poh-al-bew-min-EE-mee-ah] abnormally low blood concentration of the protein albumin

**hypoaldosteronuria** [high-poh-ahl-DAWS-ter-ohn-YUR-ee-ah] abnormally low amounts of albumin in the urine

**hypochondriac** [high-poh-KON-dree-ak] region posterior to ribs (adjective); an individual who demonstrates morbid concern for his/her health despite absence of disease (noun)

**hypochondriasis** [HIGH-poh-con-DRY-ah-sis] preoccupation with bodily sensations by a patient with fear of serious illness despite medical evidence and reassurance that she/he is not ill

**hypochromic** [high-poh-KROH-mik] containing a lower amount of pigmentation than is normal for the bodily tissue

**hypodermis** [high-poh-DER-mis] innermost skin layer

**hypogastric** [high-poh-GAS-trik] pertaining to the area below the stomach

**hypoglycemia** [high-poh-gly-SEE-mee-ah] abnormally low level of blood glucose due to either inadequate caloric intake or excess insulin production

**hypokalemia** [HIGH-poh-kah-LEE-mee-ah] abnormally low quantity of potassium ions in circulating blood

**hypokinetic dysarthria** [HIGH-poh-kih-NET-ik dis-AR-three-ah] a speech disorder characterized by difficulty with regard to pitch, volume, and expressive intonation due to disorders of the extrapyramidal motor system, such as Parkinson's disease

**hyponatremia** [high-poh-nah-TRE-mee-ah] an abnormally low level of sodium ions in the blood

**hyponychium** [high-poh-NIK-ee-um] free edge portion of the nail growing beyond the phalanx tips

**hypoparathyroidism** [high-poh-pair-ah-THIGH-rod-izm] inadequate secretion of parathyroid hormones

**hypophysis** [high-POF-ih-sis] master gland that orchestrates endocrine function of the pituitary gland

**hypopituitarism** [high-poh-pih-TOO-eh-tar-izm] reduced or inadequate function due to pathology of the pituitary gland

**hypoplasia** [high-poh-PLAYZ-ee-ah] underdevelopment of an organ or tissue, often due to a decrease in the number of cells due to atrophy or destruction of tissue rather than the general size of an organ

**hyposecretion** [high-poh-seh-KREE-shun] decreased production of a substance below normal function or systemic need

**hypospadias** [high-poh-SPAY-dee-us] congenital defect in which the urethral opening is located on the penis ventral surface in males or within the vagina in females

**hypothalamus** [high-poh-THAL-ah-mus] brain structure located inferior to the thalamus that regulates temperature, appetite, thirst, sleep, behavioral patterns, and secretions from the pituitary gland

**hypothermia** [high-poh-THER-mee-ah] reduced body temperature, significantly below 98.6°F

**hypotonic fluid** [high-poh-TAWN-ik FLOO-id] liquid that is more dilute than normal body fluid; for example, hypotonic saline solution

**hypoventilation** [high-poh-ven-tih-LAY-shun] reduced or slowed respiratory rate that produces high alveolar carbon dioxide levels

**hypovolemic shock** [high-poh-voh-LEE-mik shok] condition where the circulating blood volume is sufficiently reduced such that blood pressure is insufficient to maintain tissue perfusion

**hypoxia** [high-POK-see-ah] oxygen deprivation to the tissues; if not resolved, this progresses to anoxia

**hysterectomy** [his-ter-EK-toh-mee] surgical removal of the uterus

**hysterorrhaphy** [his-ter-OR-ah-fee] suturing of the uterus

# I

**-ia** [ee-ah] *suffix;* condition of

**-iasis** [eye-ah-sis] *suffix;* process or state of

**-iatrics** [ee-at-triks] *suffix;* treatment

**iatrogenic** [eye-AT-roh-JEN-ik] condition arising out of a treatment or procedure performed on a patient

**-iatry** [eye-ah-tree] *suffix;* medical treatment area or specialty

**-ic** [ik] *suffix*; pertaining to

**-ical** [ih-kal] *suffix*; pertaining to

**-icle** [ih-kl] *suffix*; small

**icterus** [IK-tar-us] yellow coloration of the conjunctivae which makes the sclerae also appear yellow

**idiopathic** [ID-ee-oh-PATH-ik] having no identifiable cause

**idiopathic thrombocytopenic purpura** [ID-ee-oh-PATH-ik THROM-boh-SY-toh-PEE-nik PUR-pyoo-rah] extensive bleeding into the skin and organs due to excessive destruction of platelets in the spleen because of autoimmune dysfunction; condition may be mild and transient in children and more recurrent and severe in adults

**ileal** [IL-ee-al] pertaining to the ileum

**ileotomy** [il-ee-OT-oh-mee] surgical excision of part or all of the ileum

**ileum** [IL-ee-um] a section of the small bowel responsible for the completion of digestion and absorption of food, following the jejunum, terminating in the lumen

**ileus** [IL-ee-us] gross absence of contractions in the small intestine following trauma, surgery, or intestinal obstruction

**iliac** [IL-ee-ak] pertaining to the hip bone

**iliac crest** [IL-ee-ak KREST] the most superior of the hip bones, distinguished by a broad, flaring rim

**iliopsoas muscle** [IL-ee-oh-SOH-as MUS-sel] a compound muscle comprised of the iliacus and psoas major muscles that flex the thigh

**iliotibial band syndrome** [IL-ee-oh-TIB-ee-al band SIN-drom] knee pain caused by mechanical friction of the iliotibial band across the lateral femoral epicondyle

**ilium** [IL-ee-um] the broad, splaying portion of the hip bone which joins the pubis and the ischium, forming the acetabulum

**immunization** [im-myoo-nih-ZAY-shun] a preventative measure to boost immunity of susceptible individuals by administering killed organisms or inactivated toxins

**immunoablation** [im-YOO-noe-ah-BLAY-shun] systematic and deliberate destruction of a patient's immune function, usually to prepare for organ transplantation or to treat severe autoimmune disorders

**immunocompromised** [IM-yoo-noh-COM-proh-myzd] the state of having a deficient immune response either due to a primary immune disorder or to administration of immunosuppressive agents

**immunoglobulins** [im-yoo-noh-GLOB-yoo-linz] glycoproteins produced by white blood cells that function as antibodies

**immunologist** [im-yoo-NAWL-oh-jist] one who practices the medical specialty of immunology; who diagnoses and treats patients who have autoimmune diseases, immunodeficiency diseases, cancer, or are undergoing transplantation of organs, bone marrow, or stem cells

**impedance** [im-PEE-dans] resistance of the bones of the inner ear to being set into motion as a result of sound waves

**imperforate anus** [im-PER-for-rate AYE-nus] an abnormality present at birth in which the rectum is closed, requiring immediate surgery to allow for elimination

**impetigo** [im-peh-TYE-goh] contagious skin condition caused by streptococci or staphylococci bacteria

**implanted cardioverter defibrillator** [IM-plant-id kar-dee-oh-VER-ter dee-FIB-rih-lay-tor] a surgically implanted medical device for patients with life-threatening heart arrhythmias

**impotence** [IM-poh-tens] inability to achieve or maintain an erection

**in situ** [in SIGH-too] in a contained or localized position; not extending beyond the point of origin

**inactivated vaccines** [in-AK-tiv-ayt-ed vak-SEENZ] a solution that has an infective agent that has been killed or substantially weakened and does not produce disease

**incentive spirometry** [in-SEN-tiv spy-ROM-eh-tree] a medical device used to encourage a patient to inhale and sustain inspiratory volume to exercise lungs and prevent pulmonary complications

**incision and drainage** [in-SIZH-un and DRAYN-ij] surgical procedure of cutting into tissue to drain fluid

**incisional biopsy** [in-SIZH-un-al BY-op-see] surgical removal of a small segment of the suspect lesion for microscopic examination

**incisional hernia** [in-SIZH-un-al HUR-nee-ah] protrusion of the bowel or abdominal structures occurring along the suture line of a prior surgical incision

**incontinent** [in-CON-tin-ent] inability to voluntarily control bowel movements or bladder function

**indigestion** [IN-dye-JEST-jun] discomfort of the gastrointestinal (GI) tract including heartburn, acid regurgitation, pain, nausea, and vomiting

**inductothermy** [in-DUK-toh-ther-mee] use of electromagnetic induction to artificially produce a fever in order to treat a primary pathology

**induration** [IN-du-ray-shun] an area of hardened tissue, caused by various pathological states

**infantile hypothyroidism** [IN-fan-tile high-poh-THIGH-roid-iz-um] congenital form of hypothyroidism, formally called cretinism

**infectious** [in-FEK-shus] caused by a pathogen such as virus or bacteria

**inferior** [in-FEER-ee-or] beneath or lower; as in reference to structures

**inferior mesenteric artery** [in-FEER-ee-or mes-en-TER-ik AR-ter-ee] major blood supply of the intestine

**inferior oblique muscle** [in-FEER-ee-or ob-LEEK MUS-sel] muscle that turns the eye downward and toward the midline of the visual field

**inferior rectus muscle** [in-FEER-ee-or RECK-tus MUS-sel] muscle that turns the eye downward

**inferior vena cava** [in-FEER-ee-or VEE-nah KAY-vah] large blood vessel that receives blood from the lower limbs and the pelvic and abdominal organs; structure begins at the fifth lumbar vertebra and continues anterior to the right atrium of the heart

**infiltration** [in-fil-TRAY-shun] substance being infused or passing into tissue or organ(s)

**inflammation** [in-flam-MAY-shun] the protective response of body tissues to irritation or injury

**inflammatory bowel disease (IBD)** [in-FLAM-ah-tor-ee BOW-el dis-EEZ] chronic inflammation of various parts of the small and large intestines; the cause is not known; symptoms include diarrhea, bloody stools, abdominal cramps, and fever

**infra-** [in-frah] *prefix*; under, below, or beneath

**infraspinatus bursa** [in-frah-spy-NAY-tus BUR-sah] a sheath located between the tendon of the infraspinatus muscle and the capsule of the shoulder joint

**infraspinatus muscle** [in-frah-spy-NAY-tus MUS-sel] skeletal muscle of the upper back that originates at the infraspinous fossa of the scapula and inserts at the upper edge of the humerus; when contracted, it extends and rotates the arm laterally

**inguinal** [IN-gwih-nal] pertaining to the groin

**inguinal lymph nodes** [IN-gwih-nal lymf nohdz] lymphoid tissue located in the groin area

**inguinodynia** [IN-gwi-noh-DYN-ee-uh] pain in the groin area due to trauma, space-occupying tumors, or infection

**inhalation** [in-ha-LAY-shun] the process of drawing air into the lungs

**inspection** [in-SPEK-shun] visual observation of external surfaces or internal body cavities

**inspiratory reserve volume (IRV)** [in-SPY-ra-tory ree-ZERV VOL-yoom] the volume of air entering the lungs combined with the tidal volume (TV) during forced inhalation; average value = 3,000 cc

**insulin resistance** [IN-soo-lin reh-ZIS-tans] defective use of the insulin that is produced

**insulin shock** [IN-soo-lin shok] severe hypoglycemia produced by excess insulin and inadequate food intake; characterized by diaphoresis, tremors, restlessness, confusion, diplopia, delirium, convulsions, and circulatory collapse

**integument** [in-TEG-yoo-ment] the skin; comprised of all layers: the epidermis, dermis, and corium

**inter-** [in-ter] *prefix*; between

**intercostal** [in-tur-KOS-tul] muscle group that contracts and relaxes the rib cage during respiration

**intercostal retractions** [IN-tur-KOS-tul re-TRAK-shunz] inward movement of the soft tissue between the ribs during inspiration

**intercostals** [in-tur-KOS-tul] pertaining to muscles in spaces between the ribs

**interferons (IFNs)** [in-ter-FEER-onz] antimicrobial glycoproteins produced in response to viral invasion; their presence stimulates cytotoxic T-cell activity and amplifies macrophage action

**interleukin** [in-ter-LOO-kin] collective group of multifunctional cytokines; synthesized by lymphocytes, monocytes, and macrophages

**intermittent claudication** [in-ter-MIT-ent KLAW-di-KAY-shun] condition caused by inadequate oxygen supply to the muscles; characterized by calf muscle pain and weakness triggered by walking

**internal genitalia** [in-TER-nal JEN-ih-TAL-ee-ah] sexual and reproductive organs anatomically located inside the body, including the prostate in males and the ovaries, fallopian tubes, cervix, and vagina in females

**internal jugular vein** [in-TER-nal JUG-yoo-lar vayn] the paired, bilaterally placed blood vessels of the interior neck that receive blood from the brain and superficial structures of the neck and face

**interstitial** [in-ter-STISH-al] pertaining to spaces within tissue, between cells or organs; also known as intercellular

**interstitial cystitis** [in-ter-STISH-al sis-TYE-tis] a chronic bladder condition in which the connective tissue is inflamed; related to autoimmune or allergic responses

**interstitial fluid** [in-ter-STISH-al FLOO-id] the portion of the extracellular fluid that is between the cells and outside the blood and lymphatic vessels

**interstitial nephritis** [in-ter-STISH-al nef-RYE-tis] acute or chronic inflammation of the renal intercellular tissue and tubules, possibly due to allergic response to Sulfamide or methicillin

**intervertebral disc** [in-tur-VUR-te-brul disk] fibrous tissue also known as the anulus fibrosus that surrounds the gelatinous center, called the nucleus pulposus, between the adjacent vertebrae

**intervertebral foramen** [in-tur-VUR-te-brul for-AYE-men] the large opening between the neural arch and the body of the vertebra that accommodates the spinal cord

**intima** [IN-tih-muh] inner layer; tunica interns

**intra-** [in-trah] *prefix*; within

**intra-articular fracture** [IN-tra-ar-TIK-yoo-lar FRAK-chur] breakage of bone in a fashion that extends through the cartilaginous covering of the bone into the joint space

**intracavitary therapy** [in-trah-KAV-ih-tar-ee THER-ah-pee] radiotherapy in which one or more radioactive sources are placed within a body cavity to irradiate the walls of the body cavity or proximal tissue

**intracranial pressure** [in-trah-KRAY-nee-al PRESH-sur] force exerted by brain tissue, cerebrospinal fluid, and blood within the cranial vault

**intractable seizure** [in-TRAK-tah-bul SEE-zur] seizures that are ongoing even with optimal medical management

**intradermal skin test** [in-trah-DUR-mul SKIN test] assessment of sensitivity to an antigen injected into the skin

**intranasal** [in-trah-NAY-zal] pertaining to the inside of the nose

**intraocular pressure** [IN-tra-OK-yoo-lar PRESH-sur] measurement of the force exerted within the eye by the intraocular fluid

**intravenous (IV)** [in-trah-VEE-nus] pertaining to the inside of a vein, as of a thrombus, injection, infusion, or catheter

**intravenous pyelogram** [in-trah-VEE-nus PIE-lo-gram] radiograph of the urinary tract to examine the structure and function of the renal calyces, renal pelvis, ureters, and urinary bladder using the intravenous injection of a radiopaque contrast medium

**intravesical chemotherapy** [IN-trah-VES-eh-kal KEE-moh-THER-ah-pee] instillation of chemotherapy drugs into the bladder for the purpose of killing rapidly dividing cancer cells in the bladder or kidney

**intrinsic asthma** [in-TRIN-sick AZ-muh] asthma of unknown cause

**intro-** [in-troh] *prefix*; into or within

**intussusception** [in-tus-suh-SEP-shun] telescoping of one segment of intestine into the lumen of an adjacent segment

**inversion** [in-VER-zhun] turning a body part inward

**ipsi-** [ip-see] *prefix*; same; like self

**iris** [EYE-ris] a circular tissue of the eye whose color is genetically determined

**irritable bowel syndrome (IBS)** [IR-rit-ah-bul BOW-el SIN-drom] a disorder that consists of severe spasms of cramping abdominal pain, diarrhea, bloating alternating with constipation, and excessive secretion of mucus from the colon; also known as spastic colon or raucous colitis

**ischemia** [is-KEE-mee-ah] insufficient supply of blood to tissue caused by arterial blockage

**ischemic stroke** [is-KEE-mik strok] diminished blood supply to a particular area due to an embolism or thrombosis

**islets of Langerhans** [EYE-lets uv LAHNG-er-hanz] insulin-producing cells of the pancreas

**-ism** [izm] *suffix*; condition

**iso-** [eye-soh] *prefix*; same, equal

**isometric contraction** [eye-soh-MET-rik kon-TRAK-shun] development of muscle tension with equal oppositional force

**isotonic fluid** [eye-soh-TAWN-ik FLOO-id] liquid that has the same concentration as normal body fluid

**-ist** [ist] *suffix*; person or category of agent

**isthmus** [IS-mus] narrow passage between two connecting body cavities or parts

**-ite** [ite] *suffix*; having the nature or characteristic of

**-itis** [eye-tis] *suffix*; inflammation

**-ity** [ih-tee] *suffix*; condition or state of excess

**-ium** [ee-um] *suffix*; tissue or structure

**-ize** [eyze] *suffix*; subject to

**jaundice** [JAWN-dis] yellow appearance of skin and sclera due to excess bilirubin

**jejunostomy** [JEH-joo-NOS-toh-mee] surgical insertion of a permanent feeding tube through the abdominal wall into the jejunum

**jejunum** [jeh-JOO-num] an 8-foot-long section of the small intestine

**joint** [JOYNT] an area where two bones come together; categorized into three types: suture, vertebral, and synovial

**joint capsule** [joynt CAP-sool] a fibrous layer that encases the entire joint

**juxta-** [juks-tah] *prefix*; near, close proximity

**juxtaglomerular** [juks-tah-gloh-MER-yoo-lur] smooth-muscle cells found near the afferent and efferent arterioles adjacent to the glomerulus

## K

**Kaposi sarcoma** [KAH-poh-zee sar-KOH mah] purplish-brown vascular malignancy first observed on the skin and mucous membranes, although it may become systemic; often associated with acquired immunodeficiency syndrome (AIDS)

**keloid** [KEE-loyd] elevated, firm hyperplasia with ill-defined borders; scar site

**kera-** [ker-ah] *prefix*; pertaining to the cornea or to a horny substance of the skin

**keratin** [KAIR-ah-tin] protein associated with hair and nails; oily secretion pertaining to hair follicles and sebaceous glands

**keratinization** [kair-ah-tin-ih-ZAY-shun] formation of a hard crust on the skin, often with a horny shape

**keratomileusis** [kair-ah-toh-my-LOO-sis] surgical correction of a refractive error by reshaping the deep layer of the cornea

**keratomycosis** [KAIR-ah-toh-my-KOH-sis] fungal infection of the cornea

**ketonuria** [kee-toh-NU-ree-uh] presence of excessive amounts of ketone bodies occurring as a result of uncontrolled metabolic conditions such as diabetes mellitus or starvation

**kidney** [KID-nee] one of two large, bean-shaped organs located in the flank region of the back that are responsible for filtering waste products out of the blood and for formation of urine

**-kine** [keen] *suffix*; movement

**kinesiology** [kih-nee-see-OL-oh-jee] study of the muscles and body movement

**kinesis** [kin-EE-sis] state of movement

**koilonychia** [koy-loh-NIK-ee-ah] deformation of the nail bed with thin, concave edges; often associated with iron deficient anemia; also called "spooning of the nails"

**Korsakoff syndrome** [kor-seh-KOF SIN-drom] brain damage due to nutritional deficits associated with chronic alcoholism; characterized by severe impairment of short-term memory; patient often resorts to confabulation to compensate for gaps in memory function

**Kussmaul respirations** [KOOS-mawl res-pih-RAY-shunz] air hunger; rapid and deep respirations without pause

**kwashiorkor** [kwah-shee-OR-kor] malnutrition in children caused by inadequate intake of calories and protein

**kypho-** [ky-foh] *prefix*; having a curvature or hump

**kyphoscoliosis** [KY-foh-SKOH-lee-OH-sis] a complex abnormal curvature of the spine with components of both kyphosis and scoliosis; often treated with a back brace or surgery to fuse and straighten the spine

**kyphosis** [ky-FOH-sis] abnormal and excessive posterior curvature of the thoracic spine; also known as humpback or hunchback

**kyphotic pelvis** [ky-FAWT-ik PEL-vis] abnormal backward curvature of the lumbar spine resulting in a narrowed pelvic diameter

# L

**labial** [LAY-bee-al] pertaining to the lips of the vagina or face

**labyrinthitis** [lab-rin-THY-tis] viral or bacterial infection of the semicircular canals of the inner ear, causing severe vertigo

**laceration** [LAS-er-AYE-shun] a deep, penetrating wound with clean borders of skin

**lacrimal bones** [LAK-rih-mal BONZ] small, flat bones within the eye sockets, near the lacrimal tear glands

**lacrimal sac** [LAK-rih-mal SAK] the upper section of the nasolacrimal duct that collects tears and other fluids

**lactase** [LAK-tase] enzyme excreted by the villi within the small intestine to break down the sugar lactose found in milk

**lactation** [lak-TAY-shun] production of milk by the breasts following pregnancy

**lactation amenorrhea** [lak-TAY-shun ah-men-oh-REE-ah] suppression of menses while nursing

**lacteals** [LAK-tee-alz] lymphatic capillaries in the small intestine that absorb and transport fatty acids and other fat soluble substances through the lymphatic system

**lactic dehydrogenase test** [LAK-tik dee-HIGH-droh-jen-ace test] a laboratory blood test to determine the quantity of enzymes related to muscle destruction

**lactogenesis** [lack-toh-JEN-ih-sis] production and secretion of milk from the breast

**lactose** [LAK-tohs] a disaccharide found in milk of all mammals; it is made up of the monosaccharides glucose and galactose

**-lalia** [lay-lee-ah] *suffix*; condition of speech

**laparoscope** [LAP-ar-oh-skope] use of a fiberoptic surgical device to view the inside of the body through a small incision

**large intestine** [larj in-TES-tin] large bowel, located between small intestine and anal opening, comprised of the cecum, appendix, colon, rectum, and anus

**laryngeal** [lar-IN-jee-al] pertaining to the area of the larynx

**laryngectomy** [lar-in-JEK-toh-mee] surgical removal of the larynx, often due to throat cancer

**laryngitis** [lar-in-JIGH-tis] inflammation and hoarseness of vocal cords, often due to overuse or infection

**laryngoscope** [lar-ING-goh-skope] an instrument used to visualize the larynx

**laryngotracheotomy** [LAIR-in-goh-tra-kee-OT-oh-mee] surgical removal of the larynx and upper tracheal rings, often due to advanced malignancy

**larynx** [LAR-inks] region of the throat starting at the base of the tongue and ending at the upper trachea encircled by nine musculocartilaginous rings

**laser photocoagulation** [LAY-zer foh-toh-koh-AG-yoo-LAY-shun] use of a laser to seal the retina to the tissue of the interior eye

**laser thermal keratoplasty** [LAY-zer THER-mal KER-ah-toh-plas-tee] treatment of refractive errors of the eye by heating the cornea to shrink the collagen fibers, reshape the eye, and change the angle of the cornea in relation to the focal point

**laser-assisted in situ keratomileusis (LASIK)** [LAY-zer-ah-SIS-ted in SIGH-too kair-ah-toh-my-LOO-sis] a refractive procedure to correct myopia, hyperopia, and astigmatism by creating a flap of the cornea, followed by excimer laser ablation of cornea and then replacement of the flap

**lateral** [LAT-er-al] pertaining to the side

**lateral rectus muscle** [LAT-er-al REK-tus MUS-sel] muscle that turns the eye away from the midline of the visual field

**latissimus dorsi muscle** [lah-TIS-ih-mus DOR-sigh MUS-sel] muscle that extends and abducts the upper arm

**lavage** [la-VAJ] washing out of a hollow organ using a flow of liquid

**left atrium** [left AYE-tree-um] the left upper chamber of the heart that receives oxygenated blood from the pulmonary veins

**left lung** [left lung] structure of respiration located in the left chest, comprised of the superior, middle, and inferior lobes

**left pulmonary arteries** [left PUL-mo-nair-ee AR-ter-eez] vessels that transport blood from the heart to the lungs

**left pulmonary veins** [left PUL-mo-nair-ee vaynz] vessels transporting blood from the lungs to the heart

**left ventricle** [left VEN-trik-ul] the left lower chamber of the heart that receives blood from the left atrium and pumps it out to the body through the aorta

**Legionnaire's disease** [lee-jen-AIRS dis-EEZ] a severe bacterial infection with early presentation of fever and body aches; it progresses to liver and kidney damage and possibly death

**lens** [LENZ] the crystalline structure of the eye

**-lepsy** [lep-see] *suffix*; seizure

**lesion** [LEE-zhun] structural or functional alterations

**leukocyte** [LOO-koh-sight] white blood cells including the five subtypes: lymphocytes, monocytes, neutrophils, basophils, and eosinophils; normal blood values range from 5,000 to 10,000 per cubic millimeter

**leukocytosis** [loo-koh-sy-TOH-sis] increase in the actual number of leukocytes in the blood

**leukoderma** [loo-koh-DUR-mah] loss of melanin as a result of disease

**leukoplakia** [loo-koh-PLAY-kee-ah] whitening of the epithelium

**levator ani** [le-VAY-tar AY-nigh] a muscle of the pelvic floor that supports the pelvic organs

**levo-** [lee-voh] *prefix*; left

**levoscoliosis** [LEE-voh-SKOH-lee-OH-sis] spinal curves toward the patient's left

**Lewy body dementia** [LU-ee BOD-ee dee-MEN-sha] cognitive deterioration with rapid decline, delusions, and agitation

**ligament** [LIG-ah-ment] strong, fibrous bands of connective tissue that function to hold the two bone ends to a muscle or organ

**limbic lobe** [LIM-bik lohb] an area of the brain located around the medial aspect of the cerebral hemispheres and superior to the corpus callosum that joins the hemispheres; also known as the cingulate gyrus

**limbus** [LIM-bus] transitional area of cornea where the cornea is overlapped by the sclera

**lingual** [LIN-gwal] adjective form referring to the tongue

**lingual tonsils** [LIN-gwal TAWN-silz] lymphatic tissue located on both sides of the base of the tongue in the hypopharynx

**lipase** [LYE-pase] digestive enzyme produced by the pancreas to emulsify fat globules in the duodenum

**lipocytes** [LIP-oh-sights] fat cells

**lipoma** [lye-POH-mah] benign, fatty tumor

**-lith** [lith] *suffix*; stone

**-lithesis** [lith-ee-sis] *suffix*; slipping

**lithogenesis** [LITH-oh-JEN-eh-sis] formation of a stone in the body

**lithotripsy** [lith-oh-TRIP-see] procedure to remove an embedded kidney stone through a percutaneous incision

**lithotriptor** [LITH-oh-trip-tor] instrument that generates sound waves to break up a stone in the body

**liver** [LIV-er] the largest solid organ of the body, located in the upper right abdominal area, that contains four lobes and is responsible for metabolic, excretory, and detoxification functions

**localized** [LOH-kal-eyzd] limited to a specific region or body part

**-logist** [loh-jist] *suffix*; specialist in study or treatment of a clinical area

**-logy** [loh-jee] *suffix*; study of

**long QT syndrome** [LONG kyoo-tee SIN-drom] a genetically transmitted rhythm disturbance that places children at risk for ventricular fibrillation and sudden death

**loop of Henle** [LOOP uv HEN-lee] a U-shaped segment of the renal tubule, comprised of the thin descending limb and thick ascending limb

**lordosis** [lor-DOH-sis] abnormal, excessive, anterior curvature of the lumbar spine; also known as swayback or lordotic curvature

**lumbar** [LUM-bar] pertaining to the area of the lower back between the ribs and pelvis

**lumbar puncture** [LUM-bar PUNK-chur] diagnostic procedure that entails removal of cerebral spinal fluid from the subarachnoid space

**lumbar spine** [LUM-bar spyn] the five spinal vertebrae of the lower back

**lumbosacral plexus** [lum-boh-SAY-krul PLECK-sus] spinal nerve network of the lumbar and sacral regions

**lumen** [LEW-men] space inside the tubular artery, or tube; a standardized unit of light measurement called international candles; plural is lumina

**lunate** [loo-NAYT] a crescent-shaped bone located in the proximal row of the carpus

**lungs** [LUNGZ] two bilateral, spongy, cone-shaped structures of respiration contained in the pleural cavity of the thorax

**lunula** [LOO-new-lah] white, semilunar area of nail near the root

**luteinizing hormone** [LOO-tee-ih-ny-zing HOR-mone] a hormone that stimulates interstitial cells of the testes and the corpus luteum in the ovary

**Lyme disease** [LIME dis-EEZ] arthritis caused by the bite of an infected deer tick; symptoms include a nonpruritic erythemic rash that expands outward, bull's-eye rash, joint pain, fever, chills, and fatigue

**lymph** [LIMF] fluid in the lymphatic vessels

**lymph nodes** [LIMF nohdz] small, kidney-shaped organs that contain large numbers of lymphocytes and macrophages; these nodes occur alone and in chains along the lymphatic duct

**lymph nodules** [LIMF NOD-yoolz] areas of lymphocyte formation within the lymph nodes

**lymphadenopathy** [lim-fad-eh-NOP-ah-thee] enlargement of the lymph nodes due to activation and proliferation of lymphocytes and phagocytes that is most often associated with infection or invasion of a lymph node by a tumor

**lymphadenosis** [lim-FAD-eh-NOH-sis] enlargement of the lymph nodes

**lymphangioma** [lim-FAN-jee-oh-ma] tumor made up of lymph vessels

**lymphangioplasty** [lim-FAN-jee-oh-plas-tee] establishment of artificial lymph ducts to bypass areas of blocked lymphatic circulation

**lymphangitis** [lim-fan-JIGH-tis] inflammation of the lymph vessels

**lymphatic ducts** [lim-FAH-tik dukts] channels that collect lymph from organs and regions of the body

**lymphatic system** [lim-FAH-tik SIS-tem] comprised of the main lymphatic duct, draining lymph from the upper right body quadrant and returning it to the bloodstream via the right subclavian vein

**lymphatic vessels** [lim-FAH-tik VES-selz] the efferent passage for lymph

**lymphatics** [lim-FAH-tiks] a vascular channel that transports lymph; singular is sometimes used as an adjective to describe the quality of being sluggish

**lymphocytes** [LIM-foh-sights] leukocytes (white blood cells) found in lymphatic tissue

**lymphogranuloma venereum** [LIM-foh-gran-yoo-LOH-mah ven-eh-REE-um] a sexually transmitted disease caused by the *Chlamydia* species that causes reddened, painless erosions of the genitals and rectum, followed by lymph node enlargement and fistulous tracts, obstructions, and infection of the perirectal lymph nodes

**lymphography** [lim-FOG-raf-ee] a diagnostic study in which an isotope (radioactive substance) is injected into the patient's blood, taken up by the lymphatic system, and visualized through radiographic pictures

**lymphokinesis** [LIM-foh-kin-EE-sis] circulation of lymph through the lymphatic vessels and lymph nodes

**lymphokinetic** [LIM-foh-ki-NET-ick] factors or body actions that contribute to lymph circulation; includes actions such as arterial pulses, passive compression of soft body tissues, postural changes, and skeletal muscle contractions

**lymphoma** [lim-FOH-mah] neoplasm of lymph tissue; also called malignant lymphoma

**lyo-** [ly-oh] *prefix*; loosen or dissolve

**-lysis** [ly-sis] *suffix*; to loosen, dissolve, or relieve

**-lyte** [light] *suffix*; dissolved substance

# M

**macro-** [mak-roh] *prefix*; large or elongated

**macrophage** [MAK-roh-fayj] monocyte cells that have migrated from circulation into tissues and are responsible for immune response by engulfing and ingesting foreign antigens

**macula lutea** [MAK-yoo-lah loo-TEE-ah] a yellow-colored spot visible on the retina near the optic nerve of the retina that contains the fovea centralis, which is the point of greatest visual focus

**macular degeneration** [MAK-yoo-lar dee-jen-er-AY-shun] loss of central vision due to disruption of the integrity of the retina

**macule** [MAK-yool] small, circumscribed, discolored skin lesion

**magnetic resonance imaging** [mag-NET-ik REZ-oh-nans IM-aj-ing] diagnostic imaging by use of electromagnetic radiation to visualize soft tissues of the body

**mal-** [mal] *prefix*; bad or inadequate

**malabsorption syndrome** [mal-ab-SORP-shun SIN-drom] inadequate uptake of nutrients from the digestive tract that may be associated with gastrectomy, gastric bypass, or deficiency of pancrease or lactase enzymes

**-malacia** [mah-lay-sha] *suffix*; condition of softening

**malaise** [mah-LAZE] feeling unwell, often the first sign of illness

**malalignment** [MAL-ah-LINE-ment] arrangement of bone fragments after a fracture such that they do not heal properly

**malaria** [mah-LAH-ree-ah] a febrile illness with malaise, headache, fatigue, and muscular aches due to infection by protozoa from the genus *Plasmodium*

**malignant** [mah-LIG-nant] cancer, carcinoma, endangering health or life

**malingering** [mah-LING-ger-ing] demonstrating factitious medical or psychiatric symptoms in order to get a tangible reward, such as narcotic drugs or disability payments, with the patients' awareness that they are lying and know what they want to achieve from their deceptions

**Mall formula** [mawl FOR-myoo-lah] method of calculating the age of a human embryo in days; calculated by taking the square root of the length from vertex to breech in centimeters, then multiplying by 100

**malleolus** [mal-EE-oh-lus] rounded distal projections of the distal tibia and fibula that comprise the ankle

**malrotation** [mal-roh-TAY-shun] rotation of a organ or structure in such a manner as to cut off function and/or blood supply

**maltase** [MAWL-tays] enzyme that converts maltose to glucose

**mammary** [MAM-ah-ree] pertaining to breast tissue or ducts

**mandible** [MAN-dih-bul] the bone of the lower jaw

**-mania** [MAY-nee-ah] *suffix;* indicating frenzy or a hyperexcited state

**Mantoux test** [man-TOO test] use of a four-pronged device to puncture the skin to deliver purified protein derivative from the mycobacterium tuberculosis to determine patient's exposure to tuberculosis

**manubrium** [mah-NYOO-bree-um] a triangular bone located at the most superior part of the sternum

**marasmus** [mah-RAZ-mus] chronic malnutrition caused by starvation, resulting in severe wasting of body tissues with: loss of subcutaneous fat; inelastic, wrinkled skin; loss of muscle tissue and strength; failure to grow; lethargy; and hypoproteinemia

**masseter muscle** [mas-SEE-ter MUS-sel] the muscle that closes the jaw and is used in chewing

**mast-** [mast] *prefix;* breast

**mastication** [mas-tih-KAY-shun] the process of chewing

**mastoid** [MASS-toyd] portion of the temporal bone of the skull located just behind and inferior to the ear

**mastoidectomy** [MASS-toy-DEK-toh-mee] surgical removal of the distal portion of the mastoid bone (mastoid process) and portions of the mastoid sinus; usually due to untreated otitis media

**mastopexy** [MAS-toh-peck-see] plastic surgery performed to correct drooping breasts to improve their look and form

**maxilla** [MAK-sil-ah] bone of the upper jaw

**maxillofacial** [MAK-sil-oh-FAY-shal] pertaining to the maxilla and upper face region

**meatotomy** [mee-ah-TOH-mee] enlargement of a passageway or channel by making an incision

**meatus** [ME-ayt-us] an opening or tunnel that connects internal and external surfaces

**mechanical ventilation** [meh-KAN-ih-kal ven-tih-LAY-shun] use of artificially supplied respirations using an automated respirator

**Meckel's diverticulum** [MEK-elz dy-ver-TIK-yoo-lum] a blind pouch that results when the omphalomesenteric duct, which connects the gut to the yolk sac during embryonic development, fails to atrophy

**meconium** [mee-KO-nee-um] first stool produced by newborn babies, which is characteristically greenish-black, thick, and sticky

**medial** [MEE-dee-al] going toward the middle

**medial rectus muscle** [MEE-dee-al REK-tus MUS-sel] muscle that moves the eye toward the midline

**mediastinal nodes** [med-ih-STIN-al nohdz] lymph tissue in the anterior chest

**mediastinum** [mee-dee-ah-STY-num] middle body cavity, midchest, directly above the diaphragm

**medulla** [meh-DOO-lah] innermost area of an organ or structure; for example, a lymph node or the kidney

**medulla oblongata** [meh-DOO-lah ob-long-GAH-tah] section of the brain stem that is continuous with the spinal cord

**medullary cavity** [MED-uhl-ar-ee KAV-ih-tee] the long cavity in the center of a long bone that contains yellow bone marrow

**medullary rhythmicity area** [MED-uhl-ar-ee rith-MIS-ih-tee AIR-ee-uh] brain region that regulates breathing patterns

**medulloblastoma** [meh-DOO-loh-blas-TOH-mah] a soft, infiltrating tumor of the external layer of cerebellum

**mega-** [meg-ah] prefix; large or oversized

**megacolon** [MEG-ah-koh-lon] condition of the colon with extreme dilation and hypertrophy

**megakaryocyte** [meg-ah-KAIR-ee-oh-site] a large cell normally found in the bone marrow that gives rise to platelets and has a multilobed nucleus

**-megaly** [meg-ah-lee] *suffix*; enlargement

**meibomian glands** [my-BOE-mee-an GLANZ] sebaceous glands at the edges of the eyelids that secrete sebum from their ducts

**meiosis** [my-OH-sis] division of a sex cell whereby the nucleus has 23 chromosomes

**Meissner's plexus** [MIS-nerz PLEK-sus] bundle of autonomic nerves located in the submucosa of the small intestine

**melalgia** [mel-AL-jee-ah] pain in the limbs from muscular sources

**melagra** [mel-AH-grah] pain in the limbs from neurological sources

**melanemesis** [mel-ahn-EM-eh-sis] vomitus with presence of blood in stomach contents due to bleeding ulcers

**melanoma** [mel-ah-NOH-mah] malignant tumor of melanocytes

**melatonin** [mel-ah-TOE-nin] hormone that is formed by the pineal gland and involved in circadian rhythms and bioregulation

**melena** [meh-LEE-nah] dark, tarry stools that contain digested blood due to bleeding from the esophagus or stomach

**melenic** [meh-LEH-nik] having the characteristic of dark, tarry stools

**menarche** [men-AR-kee] onset of regular menstrual cycle, with usual onset at approximately 13 years of age

**Mendelsohn maneuver** [MEN-del-son ma-NU-ver] a technique of swallowing that maintains voluntary muscular contraction for a few seconds at the highest position; used for management of swallowing disorders

**Ménière's disease** [men-YARZ dis-EEZ] a rare condition of the inner ear characterized by progressive hearing loss, sensation of pressure in the ear, tinnitus, and vertigo

**meningioma** [men-in-jee-OH-mah] a benign tumor of the coverings of the brain

**meningocele** [men-IN-goh-seel] protrusion of the meninges through bone, forming a filled cyst

**meniscus** [men-IS-kus] a crescent-shaped, fibrocartilaginous structure of the knee, acromioclavicular, and temporo-mandibular, and sternoclavicular joints

**menopause** [MEN-oh-pawz] termination of menses and ability to conceive

**menorrhagia** [men-oh-RAH-jee-ah] excessive uterine bleeding during menstruation

**menorrhea** [men-oh-REE-ah] normal menstruation

**mental scotoma** [MEN-tal sko-TOH-mah] inability to comprehend or demonstrate insight into a highly emotional subject, also known as an "emotional blind spot"

**mentum** [MEN-tum] chin

**mesenteric** [mez-en-TAIR-ik] pertaining to middle intestine attachment to the jejunum and iliac, the middle parts of the small intestine

**-meso** [mez-oh] *suffix*; middle

**meta-** [met-ah] *prefix*; change, going beyond normal development

**metabolic syndrome** [met-ah-BOL-ik SIN-drom] characteristics that increase the likelihood of development of heart disease, stroke, and diabetes whereby the individual possesses three out of five known risk factors (hypertension, abdominal obesity, elevated triglycerides, low HDL, and elevated fasting glucose)

**metabolism** [meh-TAB-oh-lih-zim] entire transformation of energy and chemicals occurring within living cells, consisting of anabolism and catabolism

**metacarpal** [MET-ah-KAR-pal] the five bones that make up the hand

**metaphysis** [met-ah-FIH-sis] portion of a bone where growth occurs, situated between the diaphysis and epiphysis

**metastasize** [met-TAS-tah-size] spreading of malignant cells to surrounding tissues and other parts of the body though the blood and lymph

**metatarsal bones** [met-ah-TAR-sal bohnz] the five long bones of the foot

**-meter** [mee-ter] *suffix;* instrument used for measurement

**metered dose inhaler** [MEE-terd dose in-HAIL-er] medical device used to deliver a specific quantity of aerosolized medication to the airway

**methicillin-resistant *Staphylococcus aureus*** [meth-ah-SIL-in-ree-SIS-tant staf-il-oh-KOK-kus ar-REE-us] clustered bacteria that are not affected by the antibiotic class of methicillin

**metopic** [mee-TOH-pik] relating to the anterior portion of the cranium or forehead

**metratonia** [mee-trah-TOH-nee-ah] atony of the uterine wall following childbirth

**metritis** [mee-TRY-tis] inflammation of the uterus

**metrorrhagia** [mee-troh-RAY-jee-ah] uterine bleeding at times other than the regular menstrual period

**-metry** [meh-tree] *suffix;* process of measurement

**micrencephaly** [my-kren-SEF-ah-lee] abnormally small size of the brain

**micro-** [my-crow] *prefix;* small

**microcytic anemia** [MY-kroh-SYT-ik ah-NEE-mee-ah] anemia where the average size of circulating erythrocytes is smaller than normal

**microgram** [MY-kro-gram] unit of measurement equaling one-millionth of a gram

**microhepatia** [my-kro-hee-PAT-ee-ah] abnormally small-sized liver

**micronodular goiter** [MY-kro-NOHD-yoo-lar GOY-tur] enlargement of the thyroid gland with small nodules that give the tissue a slightly more granular appearance than normal tissue

**microphobia** [my-kro-FOH-bee-ah] fear of germs

**micturition** [mik-too-RIH-shun] urination

**micturition syncope** [mik-too-RIH-shun SIN-koh-pee] sudden loss of consciousness during urination; most often observed in men

**midbrain** [mid-BRAYN] the middle region of the brain stem responsible for auditory and visual reflex centers

**midsagittal** [mid-SAJ-ih-tal] direction of going from front to back of body

**migraine headache** [MY-grane HED-ayk] periodic and severe pain in the head associated with vertigo, photosensitivity, scintillation, nausea, and vomiting

**Minamata disease** [min-ah-MAW-tah dis-EEZ] neurological disorder due to methyl mercury intoxication resulting from eating fish contaminated with mercury waste in the water; symptoms include peripheral sensory loss, dysarthria, tremors, ataxia, and hearing and vision loss

**miosis** [mi-OH-sis] abnormal constriction of the iris muscle to decrease the size of the pupil and limit the amount of light entering the eye; associated with stroke, head trauma, and eyedrops containing agents that deactivate acetylcholinesterase

**mitochondrion** [my-toh-KON-dree-on] a rod- or oval-shaped cytoplasmic organelle that produces energy within the cell by the production of adenosine triphosphate (ATP)

**mitosis** [my-TOH-sis] the division of cells in the body in which the 46 chromosomes in the nucleus duplicate and then split, creating two identical cells, each with 46 chromosomes

**mitral insufficiency** [MIGH-tral in-suh-FISH-en-see] faulty sealing of the bicuspid valve, causing backflow of blood into the atrium from the ventricle

**mitral stenosis** [MIGH-tral steh-NOH-sis] narrowing of the mitral valve opening, causing impaired blood flow

**mitral valve** [MIGH-tral valv] the valve closing the blood flow between the left atrium and left ventricle of the heart; also called the bicuspid valve due to having two cusps (anterior and posterior)

**mitral valve prolapse** [MIGH-tral valv PRO-laps] faulty sealing of the bicuspid valve due to chordae tendineae failure that permits backward flow of blood

**mixed hearing loss** [myxt HEER-ing loss] reduced hearing acuity due to a combination of sensorineural and conductive pathology

**Mohs surgery** [MOHZ SUR-jer-ee] microscopically controlled cancer surgery

**molluscum contagiosum** [mo-LUS-kum con-tay-gee-OH-sum] a sexually transmitted disease of the skin caused by infection with a virus from the *Poxviridae* family; typical presentation is the appearance of small, pearl-shaped epidermal growths on or around the genitals

**mono-** [mon-oh] *prefix*; single

**mononucleosis** [mon-oh-nyoo-klee-OH-sis] condition of having abnormally high numbers of mononuclear leukocytes in the blood, due to infection by the Epstein-Barr virus

**monophasia** [mon-oh-FAY-zee-ah] speech disorder characterized by the inability to state anything but one word or phrase in a repetitious fashion

**monoplegia** [mon-oh-PLEE-jee-uh] paralysis of a single limb

**monorchism** [mon-OR-kizm] condition of having only one descended testicle

**monozygotic** [mon-oh-zy-GOT-ik] twins or multiple births originating from a single zygote that separates early in development; resulting individuals have identical genetic makeup

**mora reflex** [MOR-ah REE-fleks] involuntary response in infants, present from birth to six months; when startled by noise or change in position, the arms extend and then move toward the chest

**morbidity** [mohr-BID-it-ee] sickness, or state of disease

**-morph** [morf] *suffix;* form or shape

**morphology** [mor-FAWL-oh-jee] classification of organisms by structure and form

**motile** [MOE-til] pertaining to movement

**-motor** [MOE-tor] *suffix;* something that produces movement

**mucocutaneous lymph node syndrome** [myoo-koh-kyoo-TAN-ee-us lymf nohd SIN-drom] a febrile illness in children marked by fever, rashes, lymphadenopathy, and cardiac complications; also known as Kawasaki disease

**mucolytic** [myoo-koh-LIH-tik] drug(s) used to break up thick mucus so it can be coughed up

**mucopurulent** [myoo-koh-PUR-uu-lent] mucus with pus, usually indicative of chronic obstructive pulmonary disease (COPD)

**mucosa** [myoo-KOH-sah] mucous membrane

**multi-** [mul-tie] *prefix;* many

**multi-infarct dementia** [MUL-tie-IN-farkt dee-MEN-shee-ah] decreased cognitive functioning due to many small vascular occlusions in the brain

**multipara** [mul-tih-PAR-ah] a woman who has carried more than one fetus to the point of viability

**multiple sclerosis (MS)** [MUL-tih-pul skle-ROH-sis] disease of the central nervous system characterized by the demyelination and deterioration of the myelin sheath of nerve fibers with episodes of neurological dysfunction (exacerbation) followed by recovery (remission)

**Münchhausen by proxy** [mun-CHOW-zen by PRAWX-see] patient creates illness in another person, often a child or other dependent individual, by inducing physical symptoms with drugs or by contaminating laboratory tests, in order to gain attention as the sacrificing, loving caregiver

**Münchhausen syndrome** [mun-CHOW-zen SIN-drom] patients with this disorder demonstrate factitious medical or psychiatric symptoms with awareness that they are lying, but are unaware of the underlying need for attention, resulting in numerous tests, treatments, and surgeries

**murmur** [MER-mer] abnormal blowing or roaring heart sounds heard on auscultation, caused by defective valves or chambers of the heart

**muscle biopsy** [MUS-sel BY-op-see] tissue sample taken for skeletal muscle for evaluation to assist in diagnosis of myopathy

**muscular dystrophies** [MUS-ku-lar DIS-troh-feez] hereditary diseases marked by muscle-cell degeneration

**muscular insertion** [MUS-ku-lar in-SER-shun] point of attachment to bone at the site of greatest movement; opposite of muscular origin

**muscular origin** [MUS-ku-lar OR-ih-jin] point of attachment to a stationary or nearly stationary bone of the skeleton; opposite of muscular insertion

**musculature** [MUS-kyoo-lah-tchur] the muscles of the body or the muscles in a particular part of the body

**myalgia** [migh-AL-jee-uh] muscle pain

**myasthenia gravis** [migh-as-THEEN-ee-uh GRAV-is] an immunologic neuromuscular disorder characterized by fluctuating muscular strength, poor activity tolerance, and notable weakness of the oculofacial and proximal limb muscle groups

**mycosis fungoides** [my-KOH-sis fung-GOYD-eez] cutaneous T-cell lymphoma characterized by irregular shaped nodules and plaques on the trunk that spread to lymph nodes and internal organs

**mydriasis** [mih-DRY-eh-sis] dilation of the pupil

**myelin** [MIGH-e-lin] white, fatty substance that forms the nerve sheath

**myelin sheath** [MIGH-e-lin sheath] a fatty substance surrounding some neurons that acts as an electrical insulator, increasing the speed of nerve impulse transmission

**myelitis** [migh-eh-LYE-tis] inflammation of the spinal cord

**myelocyte** [MIGH-eh-loh-site] an immature cell in the bone marrow that produces leukocytes

**myelogenous leukemia** [MIGH-eh-LAWJ-eh-nus loo-KEE-mee-ah] hematological disorder characterized by proliferation of myelopoietic cells and grossly increased numbers of immature and mature granulocytes in the blood and organs

**myelogram** [MIGH-eh-loh-gram] radiographic imagery of the spine and spinal nerves

**myelosuppression** [migh-eh-loh-su-PRESH-un] decreased production of blood cells by the bone marrow

**myocardial contusion** [migh-oh-KAR-dee-ul kon-TOO-shun] injury resulting from a strong, blunt force against the chest wall that injures the heart muscle, disrupting blood flow to areas of the heart muscle

**myocardial infarction** [migh-oh-KAR-dee-ul in-FARK-shun] necrosis of a portion of cardiac muscle caused by partial or complete occlusion of one or more coronary arteries; also known as heart attack

**myocardiorrhaphy** [migh-oh-KAR-dee-or-RAF-ee] surgical repair of the muscle of the heart by suturing

**myocarditis** [migh-oh-kar-DYE-tis] inflammation of the myocardium due to microbial infection, toxin exposure, or chronic cocaine use

**myoclonus** [MIGH-oh-KLOH-nus] rapid, intense contractions of a muscle group that is usually indicative of a central nervous system lesion

**myofascial pain syndrome** [migh-oh-FAY-shul payn SIN-drom] chronic discomfort in muscles and soft tissues surrounding joints; also known as fibromyalgia syndrome

**myofibrils** [migh-oh-FIGH-brilz] filaments in muscle cytoplasm

**myoglobin** [migh-oh-GLOH-bin] a ferrous globin complex consisting of one heme molecule containing one iron molecule attached to a single globin chain

**myopathy** [migh-OP-uth-ee] any disease of the muscles

**myopia** [migh-OH-pee-ah] refractive error of the eye resulting in inability to focus on objects at a distance; also known as nearsightedness

**myositis** [migh-oh-SIGH-tis] muscle inflammation

**myotonia** [migh-oh-TOH-nee-ah] a type of dystonia characterized by an inability to relax a muscle

**myringa** [migh-RIN-guh] tympanic membrane; also known as the eardrum

**myringotomy** [mir-ing-GOT-oh-me] surgical process of cutting into the eardrum to remove fluid from the middle ear

**myxedema** [miks-eh-DEE-mah] form of hypothyroidism which occurs in adults with decreased T4 and thyrotropin hormone production; key symptom is water retention; treatment is usually by administration of synthetic T4 levothyroxine sodium or Synthroid

# N

**narcolepsy** [NAR-koh-lep-see] a sleep disorder characterized by the frequent, sudden, uncontrollable need to sleep and by temporary muscular paralysis

**nares** [NAIR-eez] the external cartilage of the nose

**nasal** [NAY-zal] pertaining to the nose

**nasal ala** [NAY-zal AYE-lah] flared cartilage on each side of the nostril

**nasogastric tube** [nay-zoh-GAS-rik TOOBE] a small-caliber tube inserted in the nose and leading to the stomach for feeding or suctioning

**nasolacrimal duct** [NAY-soh-LAK-rih-mal DUHKT] a tube that carries tears from the lacrimal sac to the inside of the nose

**-nate** [nate] *suffix;* born

**nausea** [NAW-zee-uh] an unsettled feeling in the stomach with the urge to vomit

**navicular** [nah-VIK-yoo-lar] bones of the wrist and ankle that are shaped like a boat

**nebulizer** [NEB-yoo-lye-zur] a device used for producing fine mist for inhalation for the purpose of delivery of medications directly into the lung

**necatoriasis** [nee-ka-toe-RY-ah-sis] infestation with a parasitic hookworm

**necropsy** [NEK-rop-see] examination of a body to determine the cause of death; autopsy

**necrosis** [ne-KRO-sis] death of living cells or tissue; gangrene

**necrotizing fasciitis** [NEK-roh-ty-zing fas-ee-EYE-tis] an infection that spreads extremely rapidly and travels through tissue along superficial and deep planes; treatment includes aggressive surgical debridement and antibiotics in order to prevent death

**needle biopsy** [NEE-del BY-op-see] procedure of obtaining a deep-tissue sample for examination by piercing a lesion with a needle and withdrawing the tissue in the lumen of the needle

**negative pressure ventilation** [NEG-ah-tiv PRESH-sur ven-tih-LAY-shun] mechanical support of respiration using chambers that encase the body to create intermittent subatmospheric pressure to extend the chest outward and fill the lungs

**neo-** [nee-oh] *prefix*; new

**neologism** [nee-AWL-oh-jizm] fabricated words with meaning known only to the speaker; sometimes associated with schizophrenia or Tourette's disorder

**neoplasm** [NEE-oh-plaz-im] new growth of cells that may be malignant or benign

**neoplastic** [NEE-oh-plas-tik] pertaining to a growth of tissue which may be benign or malignant

**neoplastic heart syndrome** [NEE-oh-plas-tik hart SIN-drom] absence or stenosis of the mitral and aortic valves associated with an abnormally small left ventricle and aortic arch, possibly due to genetic factors

**nephrectomy** [nef-REK-toh-mee] surgical removal of a kidney

**nephritis** [nef-RYE-tis] inflammation of the nephrons or kidney inflammation as seen in acute nephritis, glomerulonephritis, and interstitial nephritis

**nephroblastoma** [NEF-roh-blas-TOH-mah] a rapidly developing, malignant tumor of the kidney occurring in children with deletion of chromosomes 11 and 16; also called Wilms tumor

**nephrolithotomy** [NEF-roh-lith-AWT-oh-mee] surgical procedure in which a small incision is made in the skin for the use of a fiberoptic scope to remove renal calculi

**nephropathy** [neh-FROP-ah-thee] kidney disease

**nephropexy** [NEF-roh-pek-see] surgical fixation to secure a floating or ptotic kidney

**nephroptosis** [nef-rop-TOE-sis] moveable or downward displacement of the kidney

**nephrosis** [nef-ROH-sis] degenerative renal condition characterized by damage to the renal tubules without inflammation; also called nephrotic syndrome

**nephrotic syndrome** [nef-ROT-ik SIN-drom] degenerative renal lesions resulting from damage to the basement membrane of the glomeruli; commonly seen as a complication from systemic diseases such as diabetes mellitus, systemic lupus erythematosus, and multiple myeloma

**nephrotoxic** [nef-roh-TOK-sik] poisonous or destructive to the kidney

**nerve block** [NERV blok] injection of anesthetic into peripheral nerves or nerve trunks to interrupt sensation

**nerve cell fiber** [nerv sel FY-ber] linked neurons that transmit electrical and chemical messages between the body and central nervous system

**nerve decompression** [nerv dee-kom-PRESH-un] surgical intervention to relieve pressure on a nerve by excision of constricting bands of tissue or by enlarging the bony canal

**nerve impulse** [NERV IM-puls] transmission of stimuli to or from the central nervous system

**nerve tract** [NERV trakt] a group of nerve fibers that are either afferent or efferent in their function

**nervus frontalis** [NERV-us fron-TAH-lis] branch of the occipitalis nerve that divides in the orbit into the supraorbital and supratrochlear nerves

**neural tunics** [NEW-rul TEW-niks] the layer of the eye containing the retina

**neuralgia** [nu-RAL-jee-ah] severe pain along the course of a nerve

**neurectomy** [nyoo-REK-toh-mee] partial or complete surgical excision or resection of a nerve

**neurilemma** [NU-ri-LEM-ah] membrane forming the myelin sheath

**neuroblastoma** [NYOO-roh-blas-TOH-ma] malignant neoplasm with proliferation of immature nerve cells, most often diagnosed in infants and children

**neurofibrillary tangles** [nyoor-oh-FIH-brih-lar-ee TAN-gelz] misshaped filaments on the surface of the brain associated with Alzheimer's-type dementia

**neurofibromatosis** [NU-roh-fi-broh-mah-TOH-sis] a group of genetic diseases that affect cell growth of neural tissues, with multiple subcutaneous tumors and tumors of the eighth cranial nerve

**neuroganglion** [nyoo-roh-GAN-glee-on] cysts containing fluid within a fibrous capsule attached to a tendon sheath of the hands, wrists, or feet

**neurogenic bladder** [new-roh-JEN-ik BLAD-der] urinary bladder dysfunction including incomplete emptying, urinary retention, and frequent infection resulting from impaired nervous system functioning

**neuroglia** [nyoo-ROG-lee-uh] supportive, non-nerve tissues of the peripheral and central nervous system

**neurohypophysis** [nyoo-roh-high-POF-ih-SIS] a neurological structure at the base of the hypothalamus including the infundibulum and the posterior lobe of the pituitary gland

**neuroleptic** [nyoo-roh-LEP-tik] category of pharmacological agents that treat psychotic symptoms by reducing the amount of dopamine in the brain

**neuroleptic malignant syndrome** [nyoo-roh-LEP-tik mah-LIG-nant SIN-drom] a potentially fatal complication following administration of antipsychotic medications; characterized by severe hyperthermia, confusion, gross diaphoresis, renal failure, and seizures

**neurology** [nyoo-RAWL-oh-jee] branch of medicine that deals with disorders of the central and peripheral nervous systems

**neurolysis** [nyoo-ROL-eye-is] cutting or freeing nerve tissue from inflammatory adhesions

**neuromuscular junction** [NYOO-roh-MUS-ku-lar JUNKT-shun] location of connection of nerves to muscle tissues

**neuron** [NYOO-ron] the functional unit of the nervous system responsible for conducting impulses; includes the axion, cell body, and dendrites

**neurosis** [nyoo-ROH-sis] psychiatric disorder that affects coping which results in maladaptive behaviors but does not prevent functioning

**neurosyphilis** [nyoo-roh-SIF-ih-lis] infection of the central nervous system with *Treponema pallidum*, causing dementia and other degenerative changes; may be asymptomatic or involve the meninges and vascular structures in the brain and/or spinal cord

**neurotransmitter** [nyoo-roh-TRANS-mit-er] any one of numerous chemicals that modify or result in the transmission of nerve impulses between synapses

**neutropenia** [NYOO-troh-PEE-nee-uh] condition of diminished quantity of white blood cells in the circulating blood

**neutrophil** [NYOO-troh-fil] a mature white blood cell formed in the bone marrow

**nitroglycerin** [nigh-troh-GLIS-er-in] a fast-acting vasodilator drug

**noci-** [noh-sih] *prefix*; injury; experiencing or producing pain

**nociceptor** [noh-sih-SEP-tor] a peripheral nerve responsible for perception of pain

**nodule** [NOD-uhl] a small lymph node; small circumscribed swelling

**non-** [non] *prefix*; not

**noncontributory** [non-kon-TRIB-yew-tor-ee] not involved in bringing on the condition or disease

**nondisplaced fracture** [non-dis-PLAYSD FRAK-shur] a broken bone that remains in the normal anatomical alignment

**nontoxic goiter** [non-TAWK-sik GOY-ter] thyroid enlargement without excessive production of thyroid hormone

**nonunion** [non-yoon-yun] a fractured bone that fails to heal properly

**noradrenaline** [nor-ah-DREN-ah-lin] adrenal medulla hormone; norepinephrine

**norepinephrine** [nor-ep-ih-NEF-rin] adrenal medulla hormone; noradrenaline

**normal flora** [NOR-mal FLOOR-ah] bacteria that are expected and healthy in the body

**normal sinus rhythm** [NOR-mal SY-nus RITH-em] heart rate and electrical conduction originating from the sinoatrial node

**normochromasia** [nor-moh-KRO-may-see-uh] attribute of tissues or cells that have average staining ability

**normochromic** [NOR-moh-krom-ik] pertaining to red blood cells in which the amount of hemoglobin is normal and therefore have a normal red color

**Norwood procedure** [NOR-wood pro-SEE-jur] surgical creation of a conduit between the aorta and pulmonary artery to increase blood flow to the aorta

**nosocomial** [nos-oh-KOH-mee-al] disease caused by exposure to a pathogen in the hospital setting

**nuclear scan** [nu-klee-ar skan] diagnostic technique making use of radiopharmaceutical injection, inhalation, or ingestion for the purpose of studying the structure and function of an area of the body or organ

**nuclease** [NYOO-klee-ays] an enzyme that breaks down nucleic acid

**nucleic acid** [NYOO-klee-ic AS-id] chemicals that carry genetic information in the form of deoxyribonucleic acid (DNA) and ribonucleic acid (RNA)

**nucleus pulposus** [NEW-klee-us pul-POH-sus] center of the intervertebral disc

**nulligravida** [nul-ih-GRAV-ih-dah] a woman who has never been pregnant

**nutrient foramen** [NEW-tree-ent fo-RAY-men] opening in bone through which nerves or blood vessels pass

**nystagmus** [nys-TAG-mus] involuntary rhythmic ocular movements, particularly when looking to the side; each back-and-forth motion is known as a beat

# O

**obesity** [oh-BEE-sit-tee] weight 20 percent above the recommended weight for sex and height

**obfuscation** [OB-fyoo-SKAY-shun] mental confusion associated with gross sedation and brain disorders

**obicularis oris muscle** [oh-BIK-yoo-lar-is OR-is MUS-sel] facial muscle that circles the mouth

**oblique fissure** [oh-BLEEK FISH-sur] anatomical landmark of the right lung

**oblique fracture** [oh-BLEEK FRAK-shur] a slanting-angle break in bone

**obliteration** [ob-LIT-er-AY-shun] loss of body function or part due to surgical intervention, disease, or degenerative condition

**obsession** [awb-SESH-un] constant, persistent, uncontrollable thoughts associated with anxiety and psychotic disorders

**obsessive-compulsive disorder** [awb-SESS-iv-kom-PUL-sive dis-OR-der] psychiatric illness characterized by persistent, uncontrollable thoughts that cause anxiety and compel the patient to perform excessive, repetitive activities causing incapacity

**obstetrics** [ob-STEH-triks] branch of medicine focused on the care of women during pregnancy, delivery, and the postpartum period

**obstipated** [ob-stih-PAY-ted] severe, unrelieved constipation

**obstructive cholangitis** [ob-STRUK-tiv koh-lan-JY-tis] an acute or chronic inflammation of the bile ducts due to cirrhosis or gallstones

**obstructive jaundice** [ob-STRUK-tiv JON-dis] yellowish discoloration of skin and sclera due to a gallstone or other pathology blocking the flow of bile in the bile ducts (obstructive cholangitis)

**obstructive shock** [ob-STRUK-tiv shok] condition that occurs when a blockage of the main bloodstream interferes with tissue perfusion; possible causes include compression vena cava, pericardial tamponade, and pulmonary embolism

**obtund** [ob-TUND] to dull or decrease perception of pain

**obturating embolism** [OB-too-RAY-ting EM-boh-lizm] complete occlusion of a blood vessel by a clot or plaque

**obturator foramen** [AWB-too-RAY-tor fo-RAY-men] a large opening in the ischium that is covered by a fibrous membrane and is a point of attachment for some muscles of the hip

**occipital bone** [ok-SIP-ih-tal bone] osseous formation of the posterior base of the cranium

**occipital lobe** [ok-SIP-ih-tal lohb] most distal section of the brain; involved in vision

**occipitalis muscle** [ok-SIP-it-tal-is MUS-sel] muscle that retracts and tenses scalp

**occlusion** [oh-KLOO-zhun] the action of closing off or being closed; relationship between upper and lower teeth of the jaw

**occult** [oh-KULT] hidden, not observable by the naked eye; often used in reference to bleeding in the gastrointestinal tract

**occult blood** [oh-KULT blud] hidden blood in stool that is not visible to the unaided eye

**occupational disease** [OK-yoo-PAY-shun-al diz-EEZ] health alteration due to exposure or activities associated with work activity or job

**octa-** [ok-tah] *prefix;* eight

**oculogyric crisis** [ok-yoo-loh-JYE-rik KRY-sis] acute spasm and involuntary deviation or fixation of the eyes in an upward gaze; associated with dystonia from antipsychotic or antiemetic medications

**oculomotor nerve** [OK-yoo-loh-MOH-tor nerv] the third cranial nerve, which functions primarily to send impulses to the muscles of the eyes and eyelids in order to direct movement

**oculus dexter (OD)** [OK-yoo-lus DEKS-ter] right eye

**oculus sinister (OS)** [OK-yoo-lus SIN-is-ter] left eye

**odontoid process** [oh-DON-toyd PRAW-sess] a toothlike formation on the second vertebra upon which the head rotates

**odynophagia** [oh-DIN-oh-FAY-jee-ah] difficult or painful eating or swallowing

**-oid** [oyd] *suffix;* similar to

**-ole** [ohl] *suffix*; small

**olecranon process** [oh-LEK-rah-non PRAW-sess] the curved segment of the ulna commonly referred to as the elbow

**olfaction** [ol-FAK-shun] sense of smell or act of smelling

**olfactory aura** [ol-FAK-toh-ree AW-rah] subjective sensation of smell experienced just prior to the onset of seizure activity

**olig-** [oh-lig] *prefix*; inadequate number; few; too little

**oligodipsia** [oh-lig-oh-DIP-see-uh] diminished thirst sensation

**oligopnea** [oh-li-GOP-nee-ah] infrequent breathing that causes less oxygen to enter the lungs

**oligospermia** [oh-lig-oh-SPER-mee-uh] decreased quantity of sperm in the ejaculate

**oliguria** [oh-LIG-ur-ree-ah] scant or inadequate urine production

**-ologist** [ol-oh-gist] *suffix*; one who practices a specialty

**-oma** [oh-mah] *suffix*; tumor

**omo-** [oh-mo] *prefix*; shoulder or upper arm

**omphal-** [om-fal] prefix; pertaining to navel

**omphaloceles** [oom-fal-OH-seelz] congenital malformations in which intra-abdominal contents protrude through the umbilical cord

**onch-** [onk] *prefix*; fingernails

**oncology** [on-KOL-oh-jee] a branch of medicine focused on the treatment of cancers

**onocryptosis** [on-oh-krip-TOH-sis] ingrown fingernail or toenail

**onychia** [oh-NIK-ee-ah] inflammation of the nail matrix or bed

**onycholysis** [on-ih-KOL-ih-sis] loosening of the nail from the nail bed

**onychomycosis** [on-ih-koh-migh-KOH-sis] fungal infection of the nail

**onychophagia** [on-ih-KOF-ah-jee-ah] nail-biting

**oo-** [yoo] *prefix*; ovum or egg

**oophorectomy** [oh-oof-oh-REK-toh-mee] surgical removal of one or both ovaries

**oophorocystectomy** [oh-OOF-oh-roh-sis-TEK-tom-ee] surgical removal of an ovarian cyst

**oophorragia** [oh-off-oh-RAY-jee-ah] hemorrhaging from the ovary

**open reduction and internal fixation (ORIF)** [OH-pen ree-DUK-shun and in-TER-nal fik-SAY-shun] surgical treatment to stabilize a complex fracture where an incision is made at the fracture site and the fracture is realigned using screws, nails, or plates to hold the fracture fragments in correct anatomical alignment

**ophthalmoscope** [op-THAL-moh-skop] an instrument used to examine the retina and interior structures of the eye

**-opia** [oh-pee-ah] *suffix*; condition of vision

**opiate** [OH-pee-ayt] narcotic drugs used for the treatment of pain

**opisth-** [op-isth] *prefix*; backward

**opponens pollicis muscle** [op-POH-nenz POL-ih-sis MUS-sel] muscle of the hand that pulls the thumb across the palm to enable a pinch-type grasp

**opportunistic infection** [awp-or-too-NIS-tik in-FEK-shun] disease caused by bacteria or viruses due to immunosuppression

**oppositional defiant disorder** [AWP-ih-SIH-shun-al dee-FY-ant dis-OR-der] persistent, aggressive behavior (fighting, arguing, provoking, annoying), defiance of and refusal to obey rules, disrespect for authority figures, with anger, stubbornness, and touchiness

**-opsy** [op-see] *suffix*; to view

**optic** [AWP-tik] pertaining to vision or the orbit

**optic chiasm** [AWP-tik KY-ah-zim] area in the brain where parts of the right and left optic nerves cross and join the other optic nerve

**optic disc** [AWP-tik disk] a small circular portion of the retina where the optic nerve passes through and does not have visual capacity

**optic nerve** [AWP-tik nerv] cranial nerve II, which carries nerve impulses of visual images from the rods and cones of the retina to the visual cortex in the brain

**optician** [op-TISH-an] expert who fills prescriptions for eyeglasses and contact lenses

**optometrist** [op-TOM-eh-trist] specialist in the testing of visual function and in the diagnosis and nonsurgical treatment of eye conditions

**oral antidiabetic** [OR-al AN-tee-dye-uh-BET-ik] pharmacological agents used to decrease blood glucose levels

**oral cavity** [OR-al KAV-ih-tee] the mouth, inclusive of the teeth, mucosa, and lips

**oral cholecystography** [OR-al KOH-lee-sis-TOH-grah-fee] radiological procedure that uses orally ingested tablets of radiopaque contrast dye

**orbicularis muscle** [oh-bik-yoo-LAIR-is MUS-sel] muscle that closes the eyelid

**orbicularis oculi muscle** [or-bik-yoo-LAIR-is OK-yoo-lye MUS-sel] muscle that circles the eye

**orbicularis oris muscle** [or-bik-yoo-LAIR-is OR-is MUS-sel] muscle that compresses the lips

**orbit** [OR-bit] round circuit, pertaining to the eye or bony socket in the cranium that surrounds all but the anterior portion of the eye

**orchidoplasty** [OR-kid-oh-PLAS-tee] surgical reconstruction of a testicle

**organ of Corti** [OR-gan of KOR-tee] the long, spiral-shaped structure that extends along the floor of the cochlear duct and is stimulated by sound waves

**oropharynx** [OR-oh-FAIR-inks] region of the throat located between the soft palate and the epiglottis

**-orrhea** [or-ree-ah] *suffix*; excessive discharge or flow

**-orrheixis** [or-reeks-is] *suffix*; rupture

**orthopedist** [OR-tho-PEE-dist] physician who diagnoses and treats patients with skeletal and muscular disorders

**orthopnea** [or-THOP-nee-uh] lung disease that causes the patient to assume an upright or semi-upright position in order to breathe and sleep comfortably; dyspnea and congestion in the lungs occur when lying down

**orthosis** [or-THOH-sis] orthopedic device such as a brace, splint, or collar used to immobilize or correct an orthopedic problem; often custom-made to fit the patient's specific measurements

**orthotonos** [or-THOT-oh-nus] type of tetanic spasm where the limbs, neck, and trunk are held in a rigid, straight line

**os** [OS] bone

**os calis** [os KAL-is] bone of the heel

**os pubis** [os PYOO-bis] pubic bone; one of three bones that fuse together to form the hip bone

**oscheo-** [os-kee-oh] *prefix*; pertaining to the scrotum

**-ose** [ohs] *suffix*; carbohydrate

**-osis** [oh-sis] *suffix*; condition or increased

**osmo-** [oz-moh] *prefix*; pertaining to odor, smell

**osmolarity** [oz-moh-LAIR-ih-tee] total concentration of dissolved substances in a solution; osmotic concentration

**osmotic pressure** [oz-MOT-ik PRESH-sur] part of the blood pressure that is due to plasma proteins; also known as blood colloid osmotic pressure

**osphresio-** [os-free-see-oh] *prefix*; pertaining to odor or sense of smell

**osseous** [AW-see-us] pertaining to bone

**ossicles** [AWS-ih-kulz] three tiny bones in each ear: malleus, incus, and stapes; also called the ossicular chain due to their arrangement in a row

**ossification** [AWS-ih-fih-KAY-shun] a process occurring during childhood until cartilaginous tissue is gradually replaced by bony tissue

**osteo-** [ost-ee-oh] *prefix*; pertaining to bone

**osteoarthritis** [AWS-tee-oh-ar-THRY-tis] degenerative joint disease characterized by deterioration of articular cartilage and bone hypertrophy

**osteoblast** [AWS-tee-oh-blast] mesodermal cells capable of producing new bone tissue

**osteochondrosis** [os-tee-kon-DROH-sis] degeneration and necrosis of the growth center of bones

**osteoclasis** [os-tee-oh-KLAY-sis] surgical fracture or rebreaking of a bone

**osteoclasts** [AWS-tee-oh-klasts] cells that break down areas of old or damaged bone

**osteodysplasty** [AWS-tee-oh-DIS-plas-tee] generalized skeletal dysplasia with prominent forehead and small mandible; irregular ribbon-like constrictions of the ribs and tubular bones demonstrated on x-rays

**osteogenesis imperfecta** [os-tee-oh-JEN-ee-sis im-pur-FEK-tah] brittle-bone disease characterized by sustaining multiple fractures throughout life from minimal trauma

**osteoma** [os-tee-OH-mah] a benign tumor of the bone

**osteomalacia** [os-tee-oh-mah-LAY-shee-ah] softening of the bone due to vitamin D deficiency in adults

**osteomyelitis** [AWS-tee-oh-my-LIE-tis] inflammation of the bone and bone marrow

**osteophyte** [AWS-tee-oh-fite] formation of bone fragments in the joint due to inflammation

**osteoporosis** [AWS-tee-oh-poh-ROH-sis] loss of bone structure when the rate of resorption exceeds new bone formation; results in demineralized bone that is at risk for fractures

**osteosarcoma** [OS-tee-oh-sar-KOH-mah] malignant bone tumor that occurs predominantly in adolescents and is usually located at the metaphysis of the distal femur, proximal tibia, or proximal humerus

**osteotome** [AWS-tee-oh-tohm] a surgical tool used to cut bone

**otalgia** [oh-TAL-jee-ah] earache

**otitis media** [oh-TYE-tis ME-dee-ah] inflammation of the middle ear

**oto-** [oh-toh] *prefix*; pertaining to ear or auditory function

**otolaryngologist** [oh-toh-lar-in-GAWL-oh-jist] physician who practices the specialty of ear, nose, and throat disorders; also known as ENT specialists

**-otomy** [ot-oh-mee] *suffix*; to cut or incise

**otoplasty** [OH-toh-plas-tee] surgical correction of deformities of the external ear

**otorhinolaryngology** [oh-toh-ry-noh-lar-in-GOL-oh-jee] branch of medicine focused on the function and treatment of ear, nose, and larynx disorders

**otorrhea** [oh-toh-REE-ah] discharge from the ear

**otosclerosis** [oh-toh-skle-ROH-sis] decreased function or mobility of bones of the inner ear and the oval window, causing conductive loss

**otoscope** [OH-toh-skop] an instrument that provides light and magnification for viewing the external auditory canal

**-ous** [us] *suffix*; possessing or full of; pertaining to

**oval window** [OH-val WIN-doh] opening in the temporal bone between the middle ear and the vestibule of the inner ear which is covered by the end of the stapes

**ovarian cyst** [oh-VAR-ree-an SIST] abnormal cystic growth on the ovary comprised of a closed sac containing fluid, semifluid, or solid material

**oviduct** [OH-vih-dukt] the fallopian tube

**oximeter** [ok-SIM-ee-ter] instrument used to measure the concentration of hemoglobin in the blood

**oxy-** [ok-see] *prefix*; referring to oxygen; alternate meaning: sharp, keen, acute, or pungent

**oxygenated** [OK-see-jen-ay-ted] having attached oxygen

**oxyhemoglobin** [OK-see-hee-moe-GLO-bin] oxygen molecules combine with the hemoglobin in red blood cells in the blood to form the compound oxyhemoglobin, transporting oxygen in the blood

**oxytocia** [OK-see-toh-see-ah] rapid labor

**oxytocin** [OK-see-TOH-sin] an agent that is administered to stimulate uterine contractions and accelerate delivery of a fetus

**oxytocin challenge test** [OK-see-TOH-sin CHAL-enj test] infusion of intravenous oxytocin to stimulate contractions

# P

**P wave** [PEE wayv] section of the electrocardiogram (ECG) showing atrial depolarization

**pacemaker** [PAYS-may-ker] natural or artificial regulatory mechanism of rate of an activity; often used in relation to heart contraction

**pachy-** [pak-ee] *prefix*; profuse

**pachymeningitis** [PAK-ee-men-in-JY-tis] inflammation of the dura mater of the brain

**pacing catheter** [PAY-sing KATH-eh-ter] a cardiac catheter with electrodes at the end that is inserted into the patient's right ventricle to artificially regulate heart rhythm

**Paget's disease** [PAJ-ets dis-EEZ] a disorder characterized by increased bone resorption and formation, causing thickening and softening of bones

**palinopsia** [pal-ih-NOP-see-uh] abnormal experience of recurrent visual hallucinations

**palliative care** [PAL-ee-ah-tiv kair] use of therapies intended to comfort and support those with short life expectancies, focused primarily on symptom management rather than curative goals

**pallidotomy** [pal-ih-DOT-oh-mee] surgical destruction of the globus pallidus in the brain to decrease involuntary movements associated with Parkinson's disease

**pallor** [PAL-or] unnatural lightness in color of skin due to lack of blood supply to tissue

**palmar grasp reflex** [PAL-mar grasp REE-fleks] a primitive reflex present from birth to three months of age, triggered by placing a finger across the infant's palm and eliciting a strong grip around the finger

**palpation** [pal-PAY-shun] using the fingers to touch or press on the body surface to detect masses, enlargement, edema, or tenderness

**palpebra** [PAL-peh-bra] eyelid; may be further defined as superior or inferior to denote the upper or lower lid

**palpitation** [pal-pih-TAY-shun] sensation of irregular, strong, or fluttering heartbeat in the chest or neck

**pan-** [pan] *prefix*; all

**pancolectomy** [pan-koh-LEK-toh-mee] surgical removal of the entire colon

**pancreas** [PAN-kree-as] organ with endocrine and exocrine functions

**pancreatectomy** [pan-kree-ah-TEK-toh-mee] surgical excision of part or all of the pancreas

**pancreatic islets** [PAN-kree-at-ik EYE-lets] endocrine cells of the pancreas

**pancreatitis** [pan-kree-ah-TYE-tis] inflammation of the pancreas

**pancreatography** [pan-kree-ah-TOG-rah-fee] visualization of the pancreas using endoscopy and x-rays after injection of a radiopaque contrast medium into the duct of Wirsung

**pancytopenia** [pan-sy-toh-PEE-nee-uh] gross deficiency in all components of the blood

**panic disorder** [PAN-ik dis-OR-der] sudden episodes of severe, overwhelming anxiety without an identifiable cause; patients often report feeling that they are choking or dying of a heart attack

**pant-** [pant] *prefix*; all or the whole of something

**Papanicolaou test** [pa-pa-NI-koh-lah-oo test] microscopic examination of cells scraped from the vagina and cervix after staining with Papanicolaou stain; also called Pap test

**papillary** [PAP-ih-lar-ee] small, nipple-like, raised tissue

**papilledema** [PAP-il-eh-DEE-mah] inflammation and edema of the optic disc caused by increased intracranial pressure from a brain tumor or head trauma; also known as a choked disc

**papule** [pap-YOOL] a small, raised bump or skin lesion

**para-** [pair-ah] *prefix*; beside or outside

**paracortex** [pair-ah-KOR-teks] the area of the lymph node that is rich in T-cells

**paradoxical breathing** [pair-ah-DOX-ih-kal BREE-thing] acute respiratory distress in which the chest falls and the abdomen rises on inspiration

**paralysis** [pa-RAL-ih-sis] temporary or permanent loss of motor function that may be due to stroke, spinal cord injury, tumor, or other neurological disorder

**paranasal sinuses** [pair-ah-NAY-sal SIGH-nus-ez] sinus cavities located directly adjacent to the nasal passage

**paranoia** [pair-ah-NOY-ah] a symptom of a thought disorder characterized by persistent, fearful ideas about safety that are not based on reality

**parasitic ovum** [pair-ah-SIT-ik OH-vum] the eggs of organisms, such as worms, that live within a host

**parasympathetic nervous system** [PAR-ah-sym-pah-THET-ik NERV-us SIS-tem] part of the autonomic nervous system that includes nerve fibers originating in the cranial and sacral areas and terminating in glands and muscles; function is to slow the heart and stimulate peristalsis and vasodilation to conserve or restore body resources

**parathyroid glands** [pair-ah-THIGH-royd glanz] endocrine glands on the dorsal surfaces of the lateral lobes of the thyroid gland; secretes parathyroid hormone for calcium homeostasis in the blood

**parathyroid hormone** [pair-ah-THIGH-roid HOR-mohn] substance secreted by the parathyroid gland that regulates calcium and phosphorus metabolism

**parathyroidectomy** [pair-ah-thigh-royd-EK-toh-mee] surgical removal of one or more of the parathyroid glands

**parenchyma** [pair-EN-kih-mah] parts of an organ essential to its function rather than its physical structure

**-paresis** [pair-ee-sis] *suffix;* minor weakness or paralysis

**paresthesia** [pair-es-THE-zee-ah] abnormal sensation of numbness and tingling without objective cause

**parietal lobe** [pair-RY-eh-tal lohb] the portion of the cerebrum located on the lateral and medial surfaces and covered by the parietal bone

**parietal pleura** [pair-RY-eh-tal PLOOR-ah] one of the two pleural membranes lining the thoracic cavity

**Parkinson facies** [PAR-kin-sen fay-seez] expressionless, masklike facial feature associated with Parkinson's disease

**Parkinson's disease** [par-kin-SONZ dis-EEZ] condition of slowly progressive degeneration of an area of the substantia nigra causing a decreased amount of dopamine; characterized by tremors, rigidity of muscles, and bradykinesia

**paronychia** [par-oh-NIK-ee-ah] inflammation with pus at the nail edges

**paroxysm** [PAIR-ok-sizm] sudden, recurrent symptoms of a disease

**partial seizure** [PAR-shul SEE-zure] brain dysfunction involving only limited areas of the brain with localized symptoms

**-partum** [pahr-tum] *suffix*; childbirth

**parturition** [par-tyoo-RISH-shun] labor and delivery of a fetus

**patch** [PATCH] a nonelevated skin lesion larger than 1 cm in diameter

**patella** [pah-TEL-lah] the small, rounded bone situated at the front of the knee; also known as the kneecap

**patellapexy** [pah-tel-lah-PEK-see] surgical fixation of the kneecap

**patellar reflex** [pah-TEL-lar REE-fleks] striking the patellar ligaments resulting in extension of the lower leg

**patency** [PAY-ten-see] condition of having a wide, open lumen

**patent ductus arteriosus** [PAT-unt DUK-tus ar-TEER-ee-OH-sus] the ductus arteriosus remains open after birth, allowing oxygenated blood back into the lungs through the foramen oval; characterized by thrill, fremitus, and signs of congestive heart failure

**pathogen** [PATH-oh-jen] a microorganism capable of producing disease such as bacterium, virus, or fungus

**pathogenesis** [path-oh-JEN-eh-sis] an agent that is the causative agent of a disease; for example, bacteria

**pathologic fracture** [PATH-oh-LAW-jik FRAK-shur] displacement of a bone caused by a disease process such as osteoporosis, bone cancer, or metastases

**-pathy** [path-ee] *suffix*; a disease process

**patient** [PAY-shent] one who suffers from a medical condition requiring treatment by a clinician

**patient-controlled analgesia (PCA)** [PAY-shent-kon-TROLD an-al-JEE-zee-uh] a method for administering an intravenous narcotic agent, such as morphine, using a computerized pump that permits the patient to self-administer doses of medication within preset parameters

**-pause** [pawz] *suffix*; pause or cessation

**peak expiratory flow** [PEEK eks-PIH-ra-tor-ee flow] a measurement of the volume of air after forced expiration

**pectoral girdle** [PEK-toh-ral GIR-dl] muscles of the upper chest and shoulders

**pectoralis major muscle** [PEK-toh-ral-is MAY-jur MUS-sel] the large, triangular muscle of the chest that flexes the chest and internally rotates the humerus when contracted

**pectoralis minor muscle** [PEK-toh-ral-is MY-nor MUS-sel] muscle that moves the scapula against the thorax

**pectus excavatum** [PEK-tus eks-kah-VAH-tum] a congenital deformity of the bony thorax in which the sternum, particularly the xyphoid process, is bent inward, creating a hollow depression in the anterior chest; treatment is often surgery

**pedicle** [PED-ih-kl] a bony process that extends out the back of the body of vertebrae

**pediculosis** [ped-dik-yoo-LOH-sis] skin infection caused by lice infestation; denoted by the location: head (capitis), eyelashes (palpebrarum), body (corpus), or pubis

**pedunculated polyp** [peh-DUNG-kyoo-lay-ted PAW-lip] a fleshy abnormal growth in the intestine or other tissues characterized by a thin stalk supporting a ball-shaped, irregular top

**pellagraphia** [pel-lah-GRAF-ee-uh] repetition of phrases and words in writing, indicative of brain or psychiatric pathology

**pelvic inflammatory disease (PID)** [PEL-vik in-FLAM-ah-tor-ee dis-EEZ] infection of the uterus, fallopian tubes, and adjoining structures caused by infectious agents spreading upward in the female reproductive tract, producing fever, chills, vaginal discharge, dysuria, and dyspareunia; common infectious agents are *Chlamydia trachomatis*, *Neisseria gonorrhea*, and *Escherichia coli*

**pelvis** [PEL-vis] a basin-shaped structure that includes the hip, sacrum, and coccyx of the spinal column; examples include the bony and renal pelvis

**pemphigus** [PEM-fi-gus] skin disorder with groups of bulla

**-penia** [peh-nee-ah] *suffix;* abnormal decline, deficiency

**penis** [PEE-nis] external genitalia of the male, composed of erectile tissue

**pent-** [pent] *prefix;* five

**-pepsia** [pep-see-uh] *suffix;* pertaining to digestion

**pepsin** [PEP-sin] a digestive enzyme from the stomach that breaks down food protein into large protein molecules

**pepsinogen** [pep-SYN-oh-jen] a precursor of pepsin that exists in granular form in the gastric glands

**peptic ulcer** [PEP-tik UL-sur] erosion of the upper gastrointestinal (GI) tract caused by excessive secretion of acid

**peptidase** [PEP-tih-days] digestive enzyme secreted by the small intestine that converts peptides to amino acids

**per-** [per] *prefix*; through or extremely

**percussion** [per-KUS-shun] tapping the finger of one hand, spread over a large body cavity to detect characteristics of underlying structures; use of a cupped hand to strike the chest and various lung fields in efforts to break up mucus for expectoration or suctioning

**percutaneous** [per-kyoo-TAY-nee-us] to go through the skin; used in reference to application of topical medication by friction or by insertion of a needle through the skin

**percutaneous endoscopic gastrostomy (PEG)** [per-kyoo-TAY-nee-us EN-doh-SKAW-pik gas-TRAWS-toh-mee] insertion of a permanent feeding tube through the abdominal wall using visual guidance from an endoscope passed through the mouth into the stomach

**percutaneous lithoscopy** [per-kyoo-TAY-nee-us LITH-oh-scop-ee] endoscope is inserted in a percutaneous approach into the kidney to remove a stone embedded in the renal pelvis or adjacent structures

**percutaneous transluminal coronary angioplasty** [per-kyoo-TAY-nee-us trans-LEW-mi-nul KOR-uh-nerr-ee AN-jee-oh-plas-tee] an invasive cardiac procedure in which a balloon catheter is used to restore blood flow in a blocked vessel

**perfusion** [per-FYOO-shun] passage of fluid and gases through vessels in an organ

**peri-** [pair-ee] *prefix*; around

**perianal** [pair-ee-AYE-nal] anatomical region around the anus

**pericardiocentesis** [pair-ee-kahr-dee-oh-sen-TEE-sis] drainage of the pericardial sac by a needle or catheter

**pericardium** [pair-ee-KAHR-dee-um] closed sac encircling the heart

**periodontal membrane** [per-ee-oh-DON-tal MEM-brayn] soft tissue that is immediately adjacent to the surface of a tooth and anchors it in place

**perilymph** [PER-ih-lymf] fluid found in the osseous labyrinth of the inner ear

**perimetrium** [per-ih-MEE-tree-um] outermost wall of the uterus

**perimysium** [per-ih-MIS-ee-um] the fibrous sheath that surrounds each bundle of skeletal muscle fibers

**perineal prostatectomy** [per-ih-NEE-al praw-stay-TEK-toh-mee] surgical excision of the prostate gland through the perineum

**perineorrhaphy** [per-ih-nee-OR-af-ee] suturing of the perineum, often due to a tear sustained during vaginal delivery of a fetus

**perineurium** [per-ih-NEW-ree-um] connective tissue around a bundle of nerve fibers

**periosteum** [PAIR-ee-AWS-tee-um] a thick, fibrous membrane that covers the outer surface of a bone

**peripheral nervous system** [peh-RIF-eh-tal NER-vus SIS-tem] nerves and ganglia outside the brain and spinal cord

**peripheral vascular disease** [peh-RIF-eh-tal VAS-kew-lur dis-EEZ] circulatory disorder characterized by limited or occluded small arteries and arterioles supplying the extremities

**peristalsis** [pair-ih-STAL-sis] the movement of food through the intestine via smooth-muscle contraction

**peritoneal cavity** [pair-ih-toh-NEE-al KAV-ih-tee] the space between the parietal and visceral layers of the peritoneum, used in peritoneal dialysis

**peritoneal dialysis** [pair-ih-toh-NEE-al dye-AL-ih-sis] filtration procedure that administers a dialysis solution in the peritoneal cavity to filter blood, correct electrolyte imbalances, and remove toxins, wastes, and drugs from the body

**peritoneum** [per-ih-toh-NEE-um] connective tissue that lines the abdominal cavity

**peritonitis** [pair-ih-toh-NIGH-tis] inflammation and infection of the peritoneum; this occurs when an ulcer, diverticulum, or cancerous tumor penetrates into the abdominopelvic cavity

**peritonsillar** [pair-ee-TAWN-sih-lar] tissue of the throat immediately adjacent to tonsils

**periumbilical** [pair-ee-uhm-BIL-ik-ul] abdominal area around or above the umbilicus

**pernicious** [per-NISH-us] a harmful, destructive, or fatal condition

**peroneal** [peh-roh-NEE-al] pertaining to the muscles over the fibula

**peroneus longus muscle** [peh-roh-NEE-us LON-gus MUS-sel] muscle of the anterior surface of the lower leg that extends the foot when contracted

**pertussis** [per-TUS-is] whooping cough, an infectious disease with characteristic "whoop" sound during coughing

**petechia** [pee-TEE-kee-ah] spot of hemorrhaging

**petechiae** [peh-TEE-kee-aye] pinpoint hemorrhages on the skin occurring due to platelet deficiency

**-pexy** [pek-see] *suffix;* suspension or fixation by surgical intervention

**Peyer's patches** [PY-erz PACH-ez] multiple lymphoid follicles in a compact space that form the elevations of the mucous membrane of the small intestine

**phacoemulsification** [FAY-koh-ee-MUL-sih-fih-KAY-shun] small, self-sealing incision made in the cornea, followed by an ultrasonic probe insertion to deliver sound waves to break up the lens; pieces of the lens are removed with irrigation and aspiration

**phagocyte** [FAY-goh-site] white blood cell that engulfs and digests foreign debris or particles

**phagocytic crust** [FAY-goh-sit-ik krust] cells found within the lungs that engulf debris and foreign compounds

**phagocytosis** [fay-goh-sigh-TOE-sis] the engulfing and ingesting of bacteria and old cells

**phalangeal ray** [fah-LAN-jee-al RAY] fingers in a spread-out fashion

**phalanges** [fah-LAN-jeez] bones of the fingers and toes

**pharyngeal** [fair-IN-jee-al] pertaining to the throat

**pharyngocele** [fair-IN-goh-seal] swelling or herniation of the pharynx

**pharyngospasm** [fair-IN-goh-spazm] involuntary contraction or spasm of the pharynx

**pharynx** [FAIR-inks] throat; structure through which air passes during inhalation and exhalation

**phenylalanine hydroxylose** [fen-il-AL-ah-neen hy-DROX-ee-los] an enzyme necessary to break down phenylalanine hydroxylase into tyrosine; lack of this enzyme results in excess phenylalanine in the blood that eventually spills over into the urine

**phenylketonuria** [fen-il-kee-toh-NYOO-ree-uh] a congenital disorder resulting in the inability to metabolize the amino acid phenylalanine due to the deficiency of the enzyme phenylalanine hydroxylase, causing severe neurological, skin, and psychiatric disorders; treatment consists of dietary restriction of phenylalanine

**pheochromocytoma** [fee-oh-KRO-moh-sy-TOH-ma] a tumor of functional chromaffin cells of the adrenal medulla that produces excess catecholamines, causing hypertension, nausea, headache, anxiety, and dyspnea

**-phil** [fill] *suffix*; attraction to

**-philia** [fill-ee-ah] *suffix*; attraction to

**philtrum** [FIL-trum] vertical groove in the skin of the upper lip**phimosis** [fih-MOH-sis] tightened foreskin

**phimosis** [fih-MOH-sis] tightened foreskin that cannot be retracted

**phlebitis** [flee-BYE-tis] vein inflammation

**phlebo-** [fleb-oh] *prefix*; vein

**phlebosclerosis** [FLEB-oh-skle-ROH-sis] hardening of the veins

**phlebostenosis** [FLEB-oh-sten-OH-sis] constriction or narrowing of a vein

**phlebothrombosis** [fleb-oh-throm-BOH-sis] formation of a clot in a vein resulting from inflammation

**phlebotomy** [fleh-BOHT-oh-mee] medical procedure of drawing a sample of venous blood into a vacuum tube

**phlegm** [FLEM] viscous, stringy mucus secreted by the walls of the respiratory tract

**phobia** [FOH-bee-ah] intense, unreasonable fear of a specific object or situation

**-phobia** [foh-bee-ah] *suffix*; pertaining to extreme fear

**phocomelia** [foh-ko-MEE-lee-ah] congenital malformation where hands and/or feet are directly attached to the trunk; sometimes due to prenatal exposure to thalidomide

**phono-** [foh-noh] *prefix*; voice, sound

**phorometry** [foh-RAWM-eh-tree] medical procedure to select the strength of lens that corrects the patient's refractive error and provides 20/20 vision

**photo-** [foe-toh] *prefix*; light

**photoablation** [foh-toh-ab-LAY-shun] use of a laser light to destroy or cut tissue

**photophobia** [foh-toh-FOH-bee-ah] intolerance to light

**photoreceptors** [FOH-toh-ree-SEP-torz] specialized light-sensitive cells of the eye such as rods and cones

**photorefractive keratotomy (PRK)** [foh-toh-ree-FRAK-tiv ker-ah-TOT-oh-mee] use of an excimer laser to reshape the curvature of the cornea without the creation of a corneal surface flap

**photoretinitis** [foh-toh-ret-ih-NY-tis] inflammation of the retina due to prolonged exposure to intense light

**phrenic** [FREN-ik] pertaining to the diaphragm

**phrenic nerve** [FREN-ik NERV] nerve that stimulates the diaphragm to contract, thereby initiating respiration

**phrenoplegia** [fren-oh-PLEE-jee-uh] paralysis of the diaphram

**phrenospasm** [FREN-oh-spazm] involuntary spasm or twitching of the diaphragm

**-phylaxis** [fil-ak-sis] *suffix*; protection or preventative measure

**physical therapy** [FIZ-ih-kal THAIR-ah-pee] medical interventions using active or passive exercises to improve a patient's range of motion, joint mobility, muscular strength, and balance

**physiologic anorexia** [fiz-ee-oh-LOJ-ik an-oh-REK-see-ah] decrease in appetite due to physical illness

**physiology** [fiz-ee-AWL-oh-jee] study of the function of the body

**-physis** [fih-sis] *suffix*; to grow

**pia mater** [PEE-ah MAY-ter] the vascular and innermost of the three meninges covering the brain and spinal cord

**pica** [PY-ka] eating disorder characterized by craving of nonfood items such as clay, paste, or coffee grounds

**pilonidal cyst** [py-loh-NY-dal SYST] hair that has been encapsulated in a dermal cyst

**pilosebaceous melanin** [pye-loh-se-BAY-shus MEL-ah-nin] black or dark brown pigment produced by cells called melanocytes

**pineal gland** [PYE-nee-al gland] a pinecone–shaped organ in the brain that secretes melatonin; also known as pineal body

**pinna** [PIN-nah] external structure of the ear

**pinocytosis** [PIN-oh-sy-TOH-sis] a process wherein a cell engulfs liquid by encircling the substance, forming fluid-filled vesicles

**pisiform** [PIS-ah-form] a small, pea-sized bone located in the wrist

**pituitary dwarfism** [pi-TEW-ih-tear-ee DWORF-iz-um] grossly decreased physical height; disproportion among bodily parts due to inadequate growth hormone levels

**pituitary gigantism** [pi-TEW-ih-tear-ee jye-GAN-tiz-um] excessive growth caused by hypersecretion of pituitary growth hormone, commonly due to pituitary adenoma

**pituitary gland** [pi-TEW-ih-tear-ee gland] hypophysis; so-called "master gland" that orchestrates endocrine function

**pivot joint** [PIV-ot joynt] a synovial joint in which movement is limited to rotation

**placebo** [pla-SEE-boh] an inactive substance administered in controlled research studies; when the power of suggestion is used to trigger a belief in and response to medication

**placenta** [pla-SEN-tah] the organ of fetomaternal circulatory exchange that is attached to the uterine mucosa

**-plagia** [PLAY-gee-ah] *suffix;* paralysis

**-plakia** [play-kee-uh] *suffix;* condition of forming hard deposits or plaque

**planovagus** [PLAY-no-VAY-gus] flat or flaccid longitudinal arch of the foot

**plantar fasciitis** [PLAN-tar fas-ee-EYE-tis] inflammation of the fascia in the arch of the foot, with the greatest pain at the calcaneal attachment

**plantar flexion** [PLAN-tar FLEK-shun] movement of the foot and ankle such that the toes point downward

**plantar grasp reflex** [PLAN-tar grasp REE-fleks] an automatic neurological response to stimulation of the foot that results in a curling movement as if gripping the finger; found in newborns up to eight months

**plantar reflex** [PLAN-tar REE-fleks] flexion of the foot and toes when the bottom surface of the foot is stimulated

**plantar wart** [PLAN-tar wart] viral lesion on the foot

**plaque** [PLAK] lipid deposition on the arterial wall of a vessel or structure

**-plasia** [play-zee-ah] *suffix;* growth

**-plasm** [pla-zim] *suffix;* cell or tissue substance

**plasma cells** [PLAZ-muh sellz] antibody-producing cells derived from B cells

**plasmapheresis** [PLAZ-muh-fer-EE-sis] procedure in which plasma is separated from the blood cells by rapid spinning in a centrifuge; the blood cells are returned to the donor

**plasminogen** [plaz-MIN-oh-gen] drugs that dissolve already-formed blood clots by converting plasminogen to an enzyme that breaks the fibrin strands

**-plasty** [plas-tee] *suffix;* surgical reconstruction or repair

**play therapy** [PLAY THAIR-ah-pee] use of toys and other objects to help young children express emotions or to reenact traumatic or abusive events under the guidance of a mental health professional

**pleura** [PLUR-uh] outermost membrane of the lung

**pleural effusion** [PLUR-al ee-FYOO-shun] any abnormal collection of fluid in the pleural cavity

**pleuralgia** [plur-AL-jee-ah] pain originating in the lining of the lung or the chest wall; also called intercostal neuralgia

**pleurisy** [PLUR-ih-see] inflammation of the pleura due to infection or trauma; also called pleuritis

**pleurodynia** [PLU-roh-dih-nee-ah] pain arising from inflammation or infection of the lung

**plexus** [PLEK-sus] a network of nerves, blood vessels, or lymphatic vessels throughout the body

**plica** [PLY-kah] one of the smooth folds of the synovial membrane of the joint capsule of the knee

**-pnea** [nee-ah] *suffix*; breathing

**pneumocentesis** [noo-MOH-sen-TEE-sis] surgical puncture of a lung for the purpose of removing abnormal collection of fluid

**pneumoconiosis** [new-moh-ko-nee-OH-sis] progressive lung disease caused by prolonged exposure to metallic or mineral dusts, frequently seen as an occupational exposure; symptoms include progressive lung irritation, cough, dyspnea, malaise, and frequent respiratory infections

*Pneumocystis carinii* [NOO-moh-SIS-tis kah-REE-nee-eye] an infectious microorganism that causes inflammation of the lung, formation of granulomas, and fibrosis in the bronchioles and alveoli; often associated with immunosuppressive disorders

**pneumonectomy** [NOO-mon-NEK-toh-mee] surgical removal of an entire lung, usually performed to treat lung cancer

**pneumonia** [noo-MOH-nee-ah] infection of lung; may be from bacterial or viral sources

**pneumonic plague** [nyoo-MON-ik playg] a fast-moving, often fatal infection characterized by areas of pulmonary consolidation, fevers, pain, and bloody sputum

**pneumotaxic** [new-moh-TAK-sic] area of brain that regulates or controls the respiratory rate

**pneumothorax** [noo-moh-THOR-aks] collection of air in the pleural cavity which may result in partial or complete collapse of the lung

**-poiesis** [po-ee-sis] *suffix*; to form or produce

**poliomyelitis** [POL-ee-oh-mi-LIH-tis] inflammation of the gray matter of the brain caused by a virus, often resulting in spinal and muscle deformity and paralysis

**poly-** [pawl-ee] *prefix*; many

**polyadenoma** [POL-ee-ah-den-OH-mah] malignant tumor involving many glands throughout the body

**polycystic kidney disease** [pol-ee-SIS-tik KID-nee dis-EEZ] an inherited disorder characterized by deformed nephrons that develop multiple grapelike cysts throughout the kidneys; requires dialysis and kidney transplant

**polycythemia** [POL-ee-sy-THEE-mee-uh] condition of increased numbers of red cells in the blood to increase the amount of hemoglobin available to carry oxygen

**polycythemia vera** [POL-ee-sy-THEE-mee-uh VER-ah] a chronic disorder of excessive production of red blood cells and hemoglobin concentration

**polydactyly** [PAWL-ee-DAK-tih-lee] congenital condition of having extra fingers or toes

**polydipsia** [PAWL-ee-DIP-see-ah] excessive thirst, often associated with diabetes

**polykaryocyte** [pol-ee-KAR-ee-oh-syt] cells with more than one nuclei

**polymyositis** [pawl-ee-migh-oh-SIGH-tis] autoimmune disease characterized by muscle inflammation and atrophy

**polyneuritis** [pawl-ee-nu-RIGH-tis] inflammation involving two or more nerves; often due to nutritional deficits, especially of thiamine

**polyp** [PAW-lip] small, fleshy, benign or precancerous growth that arises from the mucosa; often found in the colon and sinuses

**polypectomy** [PAWL-ih-PEK-toh-mee] surgical removal of soft, pendulous tissues from the intestine, nasal cavity, sinuses, or vocal cords

**polypeptide** [pol-ee-PEP-tyd] a substance composed of two or more amino acids

**polyphagia** [pawl-ee-FAY-jee-ah] excessive intake of food which can be due to hyperthyroidism, diabetes mellitus, or a psychiatric illness

**polypharmacy** [pol-ee-FAR-mah-see] concurrent use of multiple drugs, both with and without the knowledge of the medical team, giving rise to increased risk for drug to drug interaction

**polythelia** [pol-ee-THE-lee-uh] condition of having more than one nipple on a breast

**polyuria** [pawl-ee-YOO-ree-ah] excessive urination

**pons** [PONZ] brain tissue between the medulla and midbrain; metencephalon

**popliteal artery** [pop-LIT-ee-al AR-ter-ee] blood vessel that delivers oxygenated blood to the area of the knee and calf

**popliteal pulse** [pop-LIT-ee-al puls] a palpable throbbing movement detected at the dorsal-medial surface of the knee

**popliteus muscle** [pop-LIT-ee-us MUS-sel] muscle located behind the knee joint that flexes and assists in rotation of the thigh when flexed

**pore** [POR] a very small opening on the surface of the epithelium

**portal hepatis** [POR-tal HE-pa-tis] anatomic landmark on the liver where the portal vein, hepatic artery, hepatic ducts, and hepatic lymphatic vessels enter at the point of the transverse fissure that separates the caudate and quadrate lobes

**positive pressure ventilation** [POZ-ih-tiv PRESH-ur ven-ti-LAY-shun] a method of mechanically assisted breathing that keeps the airway open by maintaining pressure within the airway that is higher than the body surface pressure

**positron emission tomography (PET)** [POZ-ih-tron ee-MISH-shun toh-MOG-rah-fee] a diagnostic study employing computer analysis of photons detected to determine localization of metabolic and physiologic function

**post-** [pohst] *prefix*; behind or after

**post-synaptic membrane** [post-sin-AP-tik MEM-brayn] the membrane of a neuron immediately beyond the synapse

**post-synaptic receptors** [post-sin-AP-tik ree-CEP-tors] neuroreceptors located adjacent to the synapse

**posterior** [pohs-TEER-ee-or] back

**posterior chamber** [pos-TEER-ee-or CHAM-ber] thin space behind the iris

**posterior column** [pos-TEER-ee-or KOL-uhm] portion of white matter located bilaterally on the posterior surface of the spinal cord

**posterior fornix** [pos-TEER-ee-or FOR-niks] the deepest of the four recesses of the cervix

**posterior inferior vena cava** [pos-TEER-ee-or in-FEER-ee-or vee-nah kay-vuh] the primary vein that drains blood from the lower portion of the body and joins the two common iliac veins and ends at the right atrium of the heart

**posterior parathyroid** [pos-TEER-ee-or pair-uh-THIGH-royd] endocrine gland which regulates blood calcium and phosphorus ion levels by excretion of parathyroid hormone

**posteroanterior** [POS-tee-roh-an-TER-ree-or] literal meaning is "from back to front"; radiological use of term indicates passage of x-rays from back to front

**postganglionic nerve fiber** [POST-gang-lee-AWN-ik nerv FY-ber] an axon of the sympathetic and parasympathetic neuron located after the ganglionic terminus at the muscle or gland

**postictal period** [post-IK-tal PEER-ee-od] time frame following seizure activity during which the level of consciousness is decreased

**postmortem examination** [post-MOHR-tum eks-am-ih-NAY-shun] inspection of the body after death to ascertain cause of death

**postnatal** [post-NAY-tal] period of life right after birth

**postprandial** [post-PRAN-dee-ul] after a meal

**post-traumatic stress disorder (PTSD)** [POST-tra-MAT-ik STRES dis-OR-der] ongoing disabling reaction to a traumatic situation or event, with numbed emotional response, disinterest in people and current events, and repeated reliving of the traumatic event; symptoms include chronic anxiety, insomnia, irritability, and occasional violent outbursts; previously known as combat fatigue or shell shock

**postural drainage** [POS-tur-al DRAYN-ij] positioning of the body to allow for removal of mucus from the airway such that it is facilitated by the forces of gravity; often accompanied by percussion to break secretions loose

**pouch of Douglas** [POWCH uv DUG-las] the rectouterine pouch at the base of the pelvis and behind the cervix

**-prandial** [pran-dee-al] *suffix*; meal

**precancerous** [pree-KAN-ser-us] benign tissue that has potential to become malignant

**precapillary sphincters** [pree-KAP-ih-lair-ee SFINK-terz] structures between capillaries and arterioles that regulate blood flow to capillaries

**precocious puberty** [pree-KOH-shus PEW-ber-tee] reaching physical maturity at an abnormally early age

**premature atrial contractions** [pree-mah-TCHUR AYE-tree-al kon-TRAK-shuns] early cardiac beats arising from the atrium of the heart due to early depolarization of the atrium; pathology may result from ischemic or enlarged myocardium or stress, nicotine, or caffeine

**premenstrual dysphoric disorder (PMDD)** [pree-MEN-stroo-al dis-FOR-ik dis-OR-der] depressive disorder associated with the period immediately prior to the onset of the menstrual cycle, including symptoms of premenstrual syndrome (PMS) (breast, joint, and muscle pains) with depression, anxiety, tearfulness, difficulty concentrating, and sleep and eating disturbances

**prepuce** [PREE-poos] foreskin of the penis, or the skin fold around the clitoris

**presby-** [prez-bee] *prefix*; old or age-related

**presbycusis** [pres-beh-KYOO-sis] decreased hearing associated with old age

**presbyopia** [pres-bee-OH-pee-ah] loss of ability to see near objects due to aging of the lens of the eye

**pre-synaptic membrane** [pre-syn-AP-tik MEM-brayn] surface of an axon that is before the synapse

**priapism** [PRI-ah-pizm] sustained, painful erection of the penis from a pathological state

**primary follicle** [PRY-mair-ee FOL-lih-kul] structure of the ovary consisting of an immature ovum and a single layer of epithelial cells

**primary malnutrition** [PRY-mair-ee mal-new-TRI-shun] ill health that originates from lack of ability to benefit from a normally healthy diet

**pro-** [proh] *prefix*; before

**process** [PRAW-sess] prominence or projection of tissue

**procidentia** [proh-sih-DEN-shah] third-degree prolapse of the uterus and cervix, extending through the introitus

**proctocolitis** [PROK-toh-koh-LY-tis] inflammation of the rectum and colon

**prodrome** [pro-DROM] symptoms indicative of approaching disease

**progesterone** [proh-JES-ter-ohn] a steroid hormone produced by the corpus luteum that produces changes in the endometrium in preparation for implantation of a fertilized egg

**prognathism** [PROG-nath-iz-im] abnormal facial configuration in which one or both of the jaws project forward

**prognosis** [prawg-NOH-sis] predicted outcome of a disease based upon the patient's condition and the usual progression of a disease

**progressive supranuclear palsy (PSP)** [prow-GRES-iv SOO-prah-nyoo-klee-ar PAWL-zee] a progressive neurological disorder characterized by neurodegenerative changes of the basal ganglia and the brain stem; symptoms include balance difficulties, sudden falls, rigidity, bradykinesia, myoclonus, slurred speech, swallowing difficulties, and impaired ability to perform voluntary eye movements

**prolactin** [pro-LAK-tin] hormone produced by the anterior pituitary gland that stimulates breast development and lactation during pregnancy

**pronation** [proh-NAY-shun] turning of the hand or other body part downward

**pronator teres muscle** [proh-NAY-tur TEER-eez MUS-sel] muscle that functions to produce medial arm rotation

**prone** [PROHN] positioning of the body lying down, facing downward

**prophylaxis** [pro-fil-AK-sis] any measure or action taken to prevent disease

**proprioceptor** [proh-pree-oh-SEP-tor] a nerve cell that senses change in position or location of body parts

**prostate** [PRAWS-tayt] a round gland surrounding the neck of the bladder and urethra, producing fluid that becomes part of semen

**prostatectomy** [pros-tay-TEK-toh-mee] surgical excision of all or portions of the prostate gland, often by a perineal incision

**prostatic** [proh-STAT-ik] pertaining to the prostate gland

**prosthesis** [pros-THEE-sis] any medical device that replaces a bodily part or function, such as an artificial leg after an amputation

**protease** [PRO-tee-ayse] class of enzymes that breaks down protein

**protease inhibitor drug** [PROH-tee-ayse in-HIB-ih-tor druhg] one of a class of medications used to treat human immunodeficiency virus by inhibiting the ability of the virus to replicate

**proteinuria** [proh-tee-NEW-ree-ah] abnormal presence of protein in the urine

**prothrombin** [proh-THRAWM-bin] a plasma coagulation factor (factor II) synthesized in the liver

**proximal** [PRAWK-sih-mal] near the center or point of origin

**proximal flexor muscle** [PRAWK-sih-mal FLEKS-or MUS-sel] a muscle that flexes a joint

**pruritus** [prew-RYE-tus] itching

**pseud-** [sood] *prefix*; false

**pseudocyesis** [SOO-doh-sy-EE-sis] psychiatric condition where the patient has signs and symptoms of pregnancy including lack of menses, morning sickness, and weight gain, but is not actually pregnant

**pseudocyst** [SOO-doh-sist] a formation that appears to be a cyst but lacks the internal fluid-filled nature of an actual cyst

**pseudohypertrophy** [SOO-doh-HY-per-troh-fee] enlargement of muscles due to infiltration by fatty tissue

**pseudomembrane** [soo-doh-MEM-brayn] a substance that is a false layer that resembles a membrane, often occurring in the respiratory tract, making breathing difficult

**pseudophakia** [soo-doh-FAY-kee-uh] condition where the lens of the eye is replaced with connective tissue

**psoas muscle** [SOH-as MUS-sel] muscle of the internal aspect of the hip that extends from the lumbar vertebrae to the lesser trochanter of the femur; contracture causes flexion and lateral movement of the spine

**psoitis** [soh-EYE-tis] inflammation and pain in the loins originating from the psoas muscle

**psomophagia** [soh-moh-FAY-jee-ah] habitually swallowing of food without completely chewing

**psorelcosis** [soh-rel-KOH-sis] ulcerative skin lesions occurring as a result of scabies

**psoriasis** [soh-RYE-ah-sis] autoimmune skin disease characterized by white, scaly plaques

**psychiatrist** [sigh-KY-ah-trist] a physician practicing in the specialty of mental health, diagnosing and treating patients with mental illness; subspecialties include child and adolescent, geriatric, psychosomatic medicine, addiction, and forensic

**psychoanalysis** [SIGH-koh-ah-NAL-ih-sis] the oldest school of psychotherapy, developed by Sigmund Freud, in which the ideas of conscious and subconscious experiences are analyzed in a lengthy process to facilitate reintegration and development of insight

**psychologist** [sigh-KAWL-oh-jist] mental health clinician who has a doctoral degree (PhD) in psychology and provides diagnostic testing and therapy sessions for individuals and groups in psychiatric hospitals, outpatient clinics, and schools

**psychotherapy** [sigh-koh-THAIR-ah-pee] any therapy facilitated by a mental health professional which uses verbal or nonverbal communication between a patient or a group to treat a mental disorder

**psychrotherapy** [sigh-kro-THER-ah-pee] use of cold temperature to treat a disease; used in removal of skin lesions such as warts

**ptilosis** [tye-LOH-sis] loss of eyelashes due to disease or chemotherapy

**ptosis** [TOE-sis] drooping, downward placement of an organ or tissue

**ptyalism** [TYE-ah-lizm] excessive secretion of saliva; hypersalivation

**ptyalith** [TYE-ah-lith] a stone formed in the salivary gland

**ptyalocele** [tye-AL-oh-seel] a cyst formed in the salivary gland

**ptyalogogue** [tye-AL-oh-gog] pharmacological agent that causes an increase in the production of saliva

**-ptysis** [tye-sis] *suffix*; spitting

**puberty** [PYOO-ber-tee] development of genital maturity and of secondary sex characteristics, culminating in sexual maturity and ability to reproduce

**pudendal** [pyoo-DEN-dal] pertaining to female external genitalia

**puerile** [PYOO-eh-ril] concerning a child; childlike quality; used to describe lack of normal neurological or psychological functioning

**pulmonary** [PUL-moh-nair-ee] pertaining to the lungs, breathing

**pulmonary artery** [PUL-moh-nair-ee AR-ter-ee] vessel that carries deoxygenated blood from the right ventricle of the heart to the lungs for oxygenation

**pulmonary atresia** [PUL-moh-nair-ee ah-TREE-zee-ah] absence of the tricuspid or pulmonary valves

**pulmonary circuit** [PUL-moh-nair-ee SER-kut] circulation of the blood through the lungs via the pulmonary arteries and veins; transports unoxygenated blood from the right ventricle to the lungs, where the blood picks up oxygen, and then returns oxygenated blood from the lungs to the left atrium

**pulmonary function test (PFT)** [PUL-moh-nair-ee FUNK-shun test] a series of tests using diagnostic spirometry to determine lung capacities and volume

**pulmonary perfusion scan** [PUL-moh-nair-ee per-FYOO-shun skan] diagnostic study where the patient is given an injection of radioactive albumin into a vein to evaluate blood flow to the lungs using images produced by a gamma camera scanner

**pulmonary semilunar valve** [PUL-moh-nair-ee sem-ee-LEW-nur valv] valve between the heart and the pulmonary trunk

**pulmonary veins** [PUL-moh-nair-ee vaynz] vessels that carry oxygenated blood from the lungs to the heart

**pulmonary ventilation scan** [PUL-moh-nair-ee ven-tih-LAY-shun skan] diagnostic study where the patient inhales xenon gas and the images produced using a gamma camera denote the distribution of air in the lungs

**pulmonic stenosis** [pul-MOH-nik sten-OH-sis] narrowing of a valve that produces an obstruction of blood flow into the pulmonary artery, causing increased preload and right ventricular hypertrophy

**pulmonologists** [POL-moh-NAWL-oh-jists] physicians who practice in the treatment of respiratory conditions

**pulse** [PULS] a rhythmic expansion of the arterial wall in response to cardiac contraction

**pulse oximeter** [puls oks-IM-eh-ter] medical device used to measure the oxygen saturation in the tissue capillaries, using a cliplike device on the finger or earlobe

**pulse oximetry** [puls ok-SIM-eh-tree] measurement of the oxygen saturation of the blood

**pulse points** [PULS poyntz] specific anatomic locations where arterial pulsations are normally palpated, including the temporal, carotid, brachial, radial, ulnar, femoral, popliteal, posterior tibial, and dorsalis pedis

**pulse pressure** [puls PRESH-ur] difference between the systolic and diastolic blood pressure readings, which is normally ranges between 30 and 50 mm Hg

**pulverize** [PUL-ver-eyez] to reduce a hard substance to a fine powder consistency by mechanical means, often accomplished by ultrasound to break up calculi formed in the renal pelvis

**punch biopsy** [punch BY-op-see] removal of a circular piece of tissue for examination; usually performed on the cervix uteri

**punch drunk syndrome** [PUNCH drunk SIN-drom] neurological damage caused by multiple concussions resulting in functional presentation of abnormal gait and slowed movements

**pupil** [PYOO-pil] the dark center of the iris that allows light rays to enter the eye

**pupillary reflex** [PYOO-pil-air-ee REE-fleks] constriction of the iris of the eye due to stimulation with light

**pupillary response** [PYOO-pil-air-ee re-SPONS] assessment of the pupil's ability to constrict briskly and equally in response to a bright light

**Purkinje fiber** [per-KIN-jee FY-ber] cardiac muscle cell located beneath the endocardium and forming part of the electroconduction system of the heart

**purpura** [PUR-pur-ah] purple-colored, visible leakage of red blood cells into the subcutaneous tissue or mucous membranes; caused by a variety of mechanisms (trauma, clotting disorders, allergy)

**pustules** [PUS-toolz] skin elevations that contain pus

**pyelitis** [pye-eh-LYE-tis] inflammation of the kidney pelvis and calyces

**pyelocaliectasis** [PYE-ee-loh-KAL-ih-EK-tay-sis] dilation of the renal pelvis and renal calices

**pyelonephritis** [pye-eh-loh-ne-FRYE-tis] interstitial inflammation of the kidney

**pylorostenosis** [pye-LOR-oh-steh-NOH-sis] constriction or narrowing of the valve at the end of the stomach due to ulcer, disease, malignant tumor, or scarring and hypertrophy of the mucosa and submucosa

**pylorus** [pye-LOR-us] the valve at the terminus of the stomach that keeps food in the stomach, then opens to allow passage into the duodenum

**pyoderma** [pye-oh-DER-mah] any disease of the skin that produces pus

**pyothorax** [pye-oh-THOR-aks] pus in the pleural cavity, known as empyema

**pyrexia** [pye-REK-see-uh] increased temperature; fever

**pyrogen** [PYE-roh-jen] an agent, such as bacteria, viruses, or inflammatory disorders, that causes fever

**pyrosis** [pye-ROH-sis] temporary inflammation of the esophagus due to reflux of stomach acid

**pyuria** [pye-YOOR-ee-ah] presence of high numbers of white blood cells in the urine, often attributable to infection of the bladder and urethra

# Q

**QRS complex** [Q-R-S KOM-pleks] section of the electrocardiogram (ECG) showing the duration of ventricular depolarization

**quadrant** [KWAH-drant] one of four parts; for example, abdominal quadrants

**quadri-** [kwad-rih] *prefix*; four

**quadriceps muscles** [KWAH-dri-seps MUS-selz] muscle group of the anterior thigh that extends the leg; composed of recta femoris, vastus intermedius, vastus lateralis, and vastus medialis

**quadriplegia** [kwad-ri-PLEE-jee-ah] paralysis of all four limbs caused by a spinal cord lesion

**rachilysis** [ray-KIL-ih-sis] treatment of spinal curvature using pressure and traction

**rachiodynia** [ray-kee-oh-DY-nee-uh] pain in the structures of the back

**rachischisis** [rah-KIS-kih-sis] congenital condition of a spinal fissure

**rachitis** [rah-KY-tis] inflammation of the spine

**radial artery** [RAY-dee-al AR-ter-ee] blood vessel that supplies oxygenated blood to the forearm and hand

**radial pulse** [RAY-dee-al puls] bounding, throbbing sensation at the distal portion of the radius of the forearm with each contraction of the heart

**radiation therapy** [ray-dee-AYE-shun THAIR-ah-pee] use of radioactive elements as diagnostic and therapeutic interventions

**radical neck dissection** [RAD-ih-kal nek dye-SEK-shun] a surgical procedure to treat extensive cancer of the mouth and neck; includes removing parts of the jawbone, tongue, larynx, lymph nodes, and muscles of the neck

**radiculitis** [rah-dik-yoo-LY-tis] inflammation of a nerve root characterized by pain and hypersensitivity

**radioactive iodine uptake test** [ray-dee-oh-AK-tiv EYE-oh-dyne UP-tayk test] examination used to determine the rate of radioiodine absorption in the thyroid

**radioallergosorbent test (RAST)** [RAY-dee-oh-AL-er-goh-SOR-bent test] a blood test in which radioimmunoassay is used to measure the presence of IgE antibodies in the blood to detect allergies to various substances, such as certain cosmetics, animal fur, dust, and grasses

**radiocarpal joint** [RAY-dee-oh-KAR-pal joynt] the articular surface that joins the head of the radius and the bones of the wrist

**radiofrequency rhizotomy** [RAY-dee-oh-FREE-qwen-see ry-ZOH-toh-mee] procedure to relieve pain in the trigeminal nerve by use of radio waves through the skin

**radiography** [RAY-dee-oh-graf-ee] production of a shadow-type image on photographic film by exposure of film to x-rays

**radioimmunoassay** [RAY-dee-oh-im-yoo-noh-as-say] study of antigens, antibodies, enzymes, and hormones using radiolabeled reactants

**radioiodine** [ray-dee-oh-EYE-oh-dine] radioactive isotope of iodine

**radionuclide scan** [ray-dee-oh-NEW-klide skan] computer-generated images made by isolating radionuclides in the bloodstream for diagnostic purposes

**radiopharmaceutical** [RAY-dee-oh-farm-ah-sue-tic-ahl] drug containing a radioactive substance that travels to a specific body region or organ that will be scanned (i.e., CAT scan)

**radius** [RAY-dee-us] bone of the lateral forearm that is aligned with the thumb

**ramus** [RAY-mus] a branching structure from a larger anatomical structure such as a nerve or blood vessel

**Ranvier's node** [ron-vee-AYZ nohd] the nonmylenated segment of the neuron

**Raynaud's disease** [ray-NOZ dis-EEZ] a disorder characterized by numbness in fingers or toes due to intermittent constriction of arterioles

**re-** [ree] *prefix*; back or again

**rebound tenderness** [REE-bownd TEN-der-ness] reflexive, sharp pain induced by sudden release of fingers on the abdomen; indicative of peritonitis or appendicitis

**receptor** [ree-SEP-tor] a sensory nerve ending that receives a chemical message by linking or binding to a specific factor, drug, hormone, antigen, or neurotransmitter

**recession** [ree-SESH-un] the moving back or shortening of, for example, a muscle

**recovery position** [ree-KUV-er-ee po-ZIH-shun] posture used to encourage full lung expansion where the patient is placed on the left side, with the left arm extended by the left ear and the right leg crossed over the left leg

**rectocele** [REK-toh-seel] protrusion of the wall of the rectum that pushes on the adjacent wall of the vagina, causing it to collapse and partially block the vaginal canal

**rectoscope** [REK-toh-skohp] instrument used to visualize the rectum

**rectouterine pouch** [rek-toh-YOO-ter-een powch] a pocket in the abdominal pelvic cavity at the lowest gravitational point where fluids and bacteria tend to collect; also known as the pouch of Douglas

**rectum** [REK-tum] a short, straight segment of bowel connecting the sigmoid colon to the outside of the body

**rectus abdominus muscles** [REK-tus ab-DOM-ih-nus MUS-selz] paired muscles of the abdomen extending the entire length of the vertical structure of the abdomen, functioning to compress the abdominal contents

**rectus femoris muscle** [REK-tus FEM-o-ris MUS-sel] muscle of the posterior thigh

**red blood cells** [RED BLUD sellz] mature erythrocytes that contain hemoglobin

**reducible hernia** [re-DEW-si-bul HUR-nee-ah] abnormal protrusion of an organ through a wall or cavity that can be physically manipulated back into normal position

**referred pain** [ree-FERD payn] discomfort that is felt in a different location than where it originates

**reflex** [REE-fleks] an involuntary movement or action due to a particular stimulus

**reflex apnea** [REE-fleks AP-nee-uh] to gasp; sudden or temporary loss of breath

**reflux** [REE-fluks] abnormal backward flow of fluid

**refractory** [ree-FRAK-tor-ee] unable to be resolved by treatment

**refractory hypoxemia** [ree-FRAK-tor-ee hy-pok-SEE-mee-ah] lack of normal amount of oxygen in the blood that does not respond to oxygen therapy or medications

**reframing** [ree-FRAYM-ing] therapeutic communication technique that focuses on changing the emotional perspective from which an experience is interpreted

**registration** [rej-is-TRAY-shun] memory encoding or learning in the central nervous system

**regression** [rih-GRESH-shun] to move backward to a previous state of events, previous development, or primitive behavior

**regurgitation** [ree-GUR-jih-TAY-shun] the reflux of small amounts of food and acid back into the mouth

**rehabilitation** [REE-hab-il-it-TAY-shun] restoration of an individual to the highest level possible following an injury, functional loss, addiction, or incarceration

**relapse** [REE-laps] recurrence of a disease after a period of remission or recovery

**reminiscence therapy** [rem-in-is-ANS THAIR-ah-pee] psychotherapeutic technique that encourages individuals to review past pleasant experiences as a means of restoring self-esteem and personal satisfaction; this is used particularly with older adult clients

**remission** [ree-MISH-un] a period of time when symptoms of a disease are absent or greatly diminished

**renal artery** [REE-nal AR-ter-ee] paired blood vessels of the kidneys that supply oxygenated blood to the kidneys, suprarenal glands, and ureters

**renal calculi** [REE-nal KAL-kew-lye] kidney stones

**renal capsule** [REE-nal cap-sul] tissue attached immediately around the kidney and comprised of two layers: fibrous renal capsule and adipose renal capsule

**renal carcinoma** [REE-nal kahr-si-NOH-muh] cancerous tumor of the kidney

**renal colic** [REE-nal KAWL-ik] sudden, severe, sharp pain originating from the area of the back over the kidney, associated with spasms, due to presence of an embedded renal stone

**renal failure** [REE-nal FAIL-yer] malfunctioning kidneys such that they are unable to excrete wastes, concentrate urine, and conserve electrolytes; may be characterized as acute or chronic

**renal hypertension** [REE-nal high-pur-TEN-shun] elevation of blood pressure due to renal artery atherosclerosis or other kidney diseases

**renal hypoplasia** [REE-nal high-poh-PLAY-zee-ah] a kidney of small size but with normal function except that it contains nephrons of smaller size or fewer number

**renal ptosis** [REE-nal TOH-sis] kidney drop resulting from loss of supporting adipose tissue

**renal pyramid** [REE-nal PEER-ah-mid] the cone-shaped structures forming the kidney medulla

**renal transplantation** [REE-nal TRANS-plan-tay-shun] the process of placing a donor kidney into a patient

**renal vein** [REE-nal vayn] paired blood vessels of the kidneys that return deoxygenated blood from the kidneys, suprarenal glands, and ureters

**renin** [REE-nin] enzyme released by the juxtaglomerular cells when there is a drop in renal blood flow that converts angiotensin to constrict blood vessels and maintain blood pressure

**replication** [rep-lih-KAY-shun] making an identical duplicate of DNA during the early stages of mitosis or meiosis

**repression** [ree-PRESH-hun] an unconscious defense mechanism that pushes painful, traumatic events, anxiety, or guilt-producing knowledge into the subconscious, where it is dormant but able to resurface

**resection** [ree-SEK-shun] to cut out and remove

**residual volume** [REE-zid-u-AWL VOL-yoom] the volume of air that remains in the lungs at all times; average = 1,500 cc

**resocialization** [ree-sosh-al-eye-ZAY-shun] supportive measures to reintegrate a client into family and community life following a critical or long-term hospitalization

**resorption** [ree-SORP-shun] to remove by the process of absorption

**respiration** [res-pir-AYE-shun] the process of exchanging oxygen and carbon dioxide in the body; breathing movements

**respiratory center** [RES-pi-ra-tor-ee SEN-ter] a group of nerve cells in the pons and medulla that control breathing

**resting potential** [RES-ting poh-TEN-shul] base condition of the nerve due to unequal distribution of ions inside and outside the cell, typically –70 millivolts (mV)

**restless leg syndrome** [REST-less leg SIN-drom] condition of unknown etiology where the patient has the urge to move the legs to such a degree that it prevents rest and/or sleep

**restraint** [ree-STRAYNT] any method of restricting movement with cloth, belts, and other devices to prevent harm to the patient and others

**retained placenta** [re-TAYND pla-SEN-tah] failure to deliver the placenta within 30 minutes after childbirth

**retardation** [ree-tar-DAY-shun] slowed or incomplete development or function

**retention** [ree-TEN-shun] ability to recall; inability to defecate, urinate, or expel other bodily substances normally

**reticuloendothelial system** [ree-TIK-yoo-loh-en-doh-THEE-lee-ul SIS-tem] the collective, coordinated action of phagocytes in the liver, lungs, lymph nodes, and spleen that engulfs foreign substances in the body

**retina** [RET-ih-nah] membrane lining the posterior cavity of the eye that contains rods and cones

**retinaculum** [RET-ih-NAK-yoo-lum] nearly translucent band of fibrous tissue and fascia that holds the extensor and flexor tendons that cross the wrist and ankle

**retinal detachment** [RET-ih-nal dee-TACH-ment] separation of the retina from the choroid layer of the eye due to trauma, aging, or diabetes causing the blood vessels to become increasingly fragile

**retinitis pigmentosa** [RET-ih-NY-tis pig-men-TOH-sah] abnormal deposits of pigmentation behind the rods and cones, causing loss of color or night, central, or peripheral vision that may progress to blindness

**retinopathy** [ret-ih-NOP-ah-thee] any disorder that causes destruction or disruption of the function of the retina

**retinopexy** [RET-ih-noh-PEK-see] surgical procedure used to re-attach a detached retina using cryotherapy to freeze the tissue and fix all three layers (sclera, choroid, retina) together

**retinoschisis** [ret-ih-NOS-kih-sis] a split or tear in the retina of the eye

**retractions, intercostal** [re-TRAK-shunz, IN-ter-KOS-tahl] movement of the soft tissue between the ribs inward during inspiration

**retractor** [ree-TRAK-tor] a surgical instrument used to pull back tissue and structures that would otherwise obscure the view of the surgical field

**retro-** [ret-row] *prefix*; behind or backward

**retrograde** [RET-roh-grayd] movement opposite of the normal pattern, moving backward to a less developed or well state

**retrograde amnesia** [RET-roh-grayd am-NEE-zee-ah] lack of the ability to recall events before the onset of the amnesia

**retrograde pyelography** [RET-roh-grayd py-eh-LOG-ra-fee] radiological study of the kidneys, ureters, and bladder by injecting a contrast agent

**Reye syndrome** [RYE SIN-drom] a complex of symptoms following administration of aspirin for fever in children, characterized by liver damage, brain dysfunction, fever, and vomiting

**Rh factor** [arr-aitch FAK-tor] an antigen found on the surface of red blood cells called Rh-positive; absence of this antigen is indicated by the term Rh-negative

**rhabdomyolysis** [RAB-doh-my-OL-eye-sis] acute and fulminating destruction of muscle tissue; it is possibly fatal

**rhabdomyoma** [rab-doh-mih-OH-mah] a nonmalignant tumor of skeletal muscle tissue

**rhabdomyosarcoma** [rab-doh-MY-oh-sar-KOH-mah] a malignant tumor of striated muscle

**rheumatic heart** [roo-MAT-ick hart] damage to heart valves as a result of rheumatic fever

**rheumatoid arthritis** [ROO-mah-toyd arth-RIGH-tis] an acute and chronic autoimmune inflammatory disease of connective tissue that affects joints due to antibodies destroying cartilage at the articular surfaces

**rheumatologist** [ROO-mah-TAWL-oh-jist] physician who specializes in treating inflammatory and degenerative diseases of connective tissues and joints

**rhinencephalon** [ryne-en-SEF-ah-lon] anatomical portion of the cerebral cortex associated with the processing of impulses pertaining to smell

**rhinitis** [RYE-nigh-tis] inflammation of the nasal mucous membrane

**rhinophyma** [rye-noh-FYE-mah] form of rosacea affecting the nose

**rhinoplasty** [RHIN-oh-plas-tee] surgical repair of the nose to correct a defect or to change its appearance

**rhinorrhagia** [RHIN-or-rhaj-ee-ah] profuse bleeding from the nose

**rhinorrhea** [RHIN-or-ree-uh] discharge from the mucous membrane of the nose

**rhinovirus** [RYE-noh-vy-rus] a large group of viruses that cause upper respiratory infections

**rhizotomy** [rye-ZAW-toh-mee] incision in a spinal nerve root to relieve intractable pain

**rhodopsin** [roh-DOP-sin] red pigment of the rods which is bleached by daylight

**rhomboideus muscle** [rom-BOY-dee-us MUS-sel] muscle that raises and adducts the scapula

**rhonchus** [RONK-us] harsh, rattling, or whistling sound in lung fields

**rhythm** [RITH-em] the relative measurement of an impulse or activity in relation to time; regularity of action

**rib cage** [rib kayg] the bony structure of the thoracic skeleton that is formed by the 12 arched pairs of bone that insert on the sternum

**rickets** [RIK-etz] childhood disease caused by inadequate vitamin D intake

**right atrioventricular valve** [rite ay-tree-oh-ven-TRIK-yoo-ler valv] valve between the right ventricle and the right atrium; tricuspid valve

**right atrium** [rite AYE-tree-um] upper chamber of the heart that receives deoxygenated blood from the entire body except the lungs

**right coronary artery** [rite KOR-uh-nerr-ee AR-ter-ee] artery supplying blood to the heart tissue

**right lung** [rite lung] structure of respiration located in the right chest and comprised of the superior and inferior lobes

**right ventricle** [rite VEN-trih-kul] lower chamber of the heart that receives blood from the right atrium and pumps it out to the lungs by way of the pulmonary artery

**rima** [RYE-ma] cleft or fissure

**Rinne test** [RIN-ee test] a method to assess hearing by air conduction by holding a vibrating tuning fork at the base of the mastoid process and the prongs near the ear; normally, patients hear the sound longer by air conduction

**ritual** [RIH-choo-al] a detailed, prescribed order of actions; may be religious, personal, or part of psychiatric disorders such as obsessive compulsive disorder

**rod** [RAWD] light-sensitive cell; sensitive to all levels of light but not to color

**Romberg's sign** [RAWM-bergs sighn] assessing equilibrium by having a patient stand with the feet together and the eyes closed to check for swaying or falling to one side; indicates a loss of balance and inner-ear dysfunction

**rongeur** [rawn-GHER] a forceps that is used to remove small bone fragments

**root** [ROOT] a firm structural attachment, often the lowest part of an organ

**Rorschach test** [ROAR-shahk test] a psychological examination in which a patient is shown cards with abstract shapes and asked to describe what the shape of the inkblot represents; also known as the "inkblot test"

**rosacea** [roh-ZAY-shee-uh] chronic, noninfectious skin disorder marked by redness on the cheeks, nose, and chin

**rosaceiform** [roh-ZAY-shee-ih-form] the red mask appearance of cheeks, nose, and skin; typical of rosacea

**roseola** [ROZ-ee-oh-lah] a rose- or red-colored rash

**rotation** [roh-TAY-shun] one of the basic movements of a joint; having a quality of turning around an axis

**rotator cuff** [ROH-tay-tor kuff] collection of muscles that rotate the arm; includes supraspinatus, infraspinatus, teres minor, and subscapularis muscles

**rotator cuff tendonitis** [ROH-tay-tor kuff ten-don-EYE-tis] inflammation of the tendons of the supraspinatus, infraspinatus, teres minor, or subscapular muscles of the shoulder

**round ligament** [rownd LIG-ah-ment] residual structures of the umbilical vein found in the liver; a fibromuscular attachment that attaches to the uterus

**round window** [rownd WIN-doe] a circular, membrane-covered opening in the medial wall of the middle ear leading into the cochlea

**Roux-en-Y gastric bypass** [roks-en-why GAS-trik BY-pass] surgical treatment of morbid obesity by attaching the jejunum to a surgically reduced stomach pouch and connecting the bypassed duodenum to the pylorus, resulting in decreased gastric capacity and reduced absorption of food

**Rovsing's sign** [ROV-singz sighn] clinical finding indicating appendicitis whereby pressure in the lower left quadrant of the abdomen produces pain in the lower right quadrant

**-rrhage** [raj] *suffix*; sudden outpouring of drainage

**-rrhagia** [raj-ee-ah] *suffix*; sudden outpouring of drainage

**-rrhaphy** [rah-fee] *suffix*; to suture or sew together

**-rrhea** [ree-uh] *suffix*; discharge

**-rrheic** [ree-ik] *suffix*; pertaining to discharge

**-rrhexis** [rex-is] *suffix*; rupture

**rubella** [roo-BEL-ah] viral infection; also known as German measles

**rubeola** [roo-bee-OH-lah] red measles

**rubor** [ROO-bor] redness which is often associated with infection or inflammation

**rugae** [ROO-gay] folds and ridges of tissue present in mucous membranes of organs such as the intestine and vagina

**rupture** [RUP-shur] a tear, break, or protrusion of an organ or body tissue

## S

**S1** [ess-wun] sound of the heart produced by the closure of the two atrioventricular valves at the start of systole; "lub" sound

**S2** [ess-too] sound of the heart produced by the closure of the two semilunar valves at the end of systole; "dub" sound

**sacrum** [SAY-krum] a group of five fused vertebrae that are not individually numbered, except for the first sacral vertebra (S1); it joins with the hip bones to form the most posterior part of the pelvis

**saddle joint** [SAD-el JOYNT] articular surface where double motion is due to the concave surface of one joint interacting with the convex surface of another; for example, the carpal and metacarpal of the thumb

**saline solution** [SAY-leen soh-LOO-shun] an isotonic liquid preparation of salt and distilled water used for infusion or irrigation

**saliva** [sah-LY-vah] liquid that is secreted by the salivary glands and contains amylase, an enzyme that begins the process of digestion in the oral cavity

**salivary amylase** [SAL-ih-var-ee AM-ih-lays] an enzyme found in saliva that breaks down starch into simple sugars; produced by the salivary glands

**salivary glands** [SAL-ih-var-ee glanz] a group of bilaterally located glands (parotid, submandibular, and sublingual) that produce saliva

**salpingo-oophorectomy** [sal-PING-oh-oof-oh-REK-toh-mee] surgical excision of the fallopian tubes and ovaries

**salpingopexy** [sal-ping-oh-PEK-see] surgical fixation of a fallopian tube

**-salpinx** [sal-pinks] *suffix*; pertaining to the fallopian tube

**sarcoidosis** [sar-koyd-OH-sis] fibrous invasion by granulomatous tissue in the lungs, skin, lymph nodes, spleen, and parotid glands

**sarcolemma** [sar-koh-LEM-ah] sheath surrounding muscle cell

**-sarcoma** [sar-koh-ma] *suffix*; a malignant tumor

**sarcomeres** [SAR-koh-meers] contractile segment of skeletal muscle tissue

**sarcoplasm** [SAR-koh-plaz-um] intercellular material of the cell, particularly striated muscle cells

**sarcosis** [sar-KOH-sis] an abnormal formation of skin

**sartorius muscle** [sar-TOH-ree-us MUS-sel] muscle that flexes the knee and rotates the hip

**sartorius quadriceps femoris muscle** [sah-TOR-ee-us KWAD-rih-seps FEM-or-is MUS-sel] muscle of the inner thigh that abducts the leg when contracted

**scabies** [SKAY-beez] mite infection of skin characterized by a pruritic rash due to burrowing habit of the mites

**scapula** [SKAP-yoo-lah] the large triangular bone of the posterior shoulder; plural is scapulae

**scapulodynia** [skap-yoo-loh-DIN-ee-ah] painful and inflamed shoulder muscles from injury or overuse

**scapulohumeral joint** [SKAP-yoo-loh-HEW-mur-ul JOYNT] articular surface between the scapula and humerus; shoulder joint

**-schisis** [ski-sis] *suffix*; fissure or split

**schizophrenia** [SKIZ-oh-FREE-nee-ah] a major psychiatric disorder with chronic loss of connection with reality in most or all aspects of life; includes bizarre behavior, disrupted thought processes, hallucinations and delusions of persecution, and alterations in speech

**Schwann cell** [SHWAN sel] a structure of the peripheral nervous system that forms the myelin sheath and neurilemma of a nerve fiber

**sciatica** [si-AT-ih-kah] pain that follows the pathway of the sciatic nerve, caused by compression or trauma of the nerve or its roots

**scintigram** [SIN-teh-gram] nuclear image known as a 3f scintigraphy x-ray

**scintigraphy** [sin-TIG-rah-fee] injection of a radioactive tracer followed by imagery to detect areas of pathology such as arthritis, fracture, osteomyelitis, or cancerous tumors of the bone

**sclera** [SKLEER-ah] tough connective tissue that forms a white, continuous layer around the eyeball, functioning to protect the internal structures; plural is sclerae

**scleral buckle** [SKLEER-ul BUK-kel] a surgically placed band of silicone that acts to permanently tighten the retina

**scleredema** [skler-eh-DE-mah] edema and redness of the skin that precedes an acute skin infection

**scleroderma** [skler-oh-DER-mah] a chronic and progressive hardening of skin and connective tissues that produces generalized edema and limitation in movements

**scoliosis** [SKOH-lee-OH-sis] an abnormal lateral curvature of the spine with the original curve and a secondary compensatory curve in the opposite direction

**-scope** [skohp] *suffix*; instrument for examination

**-scopy** [skop-ee] *suffix*; examination

**scotoma** [skoh-TOH-mah] a blind spot in the visual field due to a variety of causes such as glaucoma, diabetic retinopathy, or macular degeneration as nerves are destroyed

**scrotal** [SKROH-tal] bag; scrotum

**scrotum** [SKROH-tum] a soft pouch of skin behind the penis containing the testes and part of the spermatic cords

**seasonal affective disorder (SAD)** [SEE-son-al ah-FEK-tiv dis-OR-der] depression due to hypersecretion of melatonin from the pineal gland in the brain due to decreased intensity and quantity of light during winter months; results in depressed mood, weight gain, and altered sleeping habits

**sebaceous cysts** [se-BAY-shus SISTS] fluid-filled sebaceous glands

**sebaceous glands** [se-BAY-shus glanz] structures that secrete sebum to the skin surface

**seborrhea** [seb-oh-REE-ah] excessive excretion of sebum from the sebaceous glands of the skin

**seborrheic dermatitis** [seb-oh-REE-ik der-mah-TYE-tis] inflammation of the sebaceous glands of the skin

**seborrheic keratosis** [seb-oh-REE-ik kair-ah-TOH-sis] benign purple-brown skin tumor(s)

**seborrheic warts** [seb-or-REE-ik wartz] pigmented skin with a greasy, raised, crusty appearance

**second cranial nerve** [SEC-ond KRAY-nee-ul nerv] the optic (II) nerve that carries impulses to the brain to deliver input for the sensory function of vision

**second-degree burn** [SEC-ond-deh-GREE burn] damage to the epidermal and dermal layers

**seizure** [SEE-zhur] sudden, transient electrical disturbances in the brain resulting from abnormal firing of nerve impulses which may or may not be associated with convulsions

**seizure threshold** [SEE-zur THRESH-old] level of neurological activity or stimulation that triggers seizure activity

**selective serotonin reuptake inhibitors (SSRI)** [seh-LEK-tiv ser-oh-TON-in ree-UP-tayk in-HIB-ih-tors] class of antidepressant medications that block the neuronal reuptake of serotonin

**semicircular canals** [sem-ih-SIR-kyoo-lar kah-NALZ] half-circle-shaped structures within the bony labyrinth of the inner ear that are critical to maintaining balance

**semicomatose** [sem-ee-KOH-mah-tohs] a state near loss of consciousness from which the patient can be aroused

**semi-Fowler position** [SEH-mee-FOW-ler poe-ZIH-shun] placement of a patient with the head of the bed elevated at least 30 degrees

**semilunar bone** [sem-ee-LEW-nar bohn] a crescent-shaped bone of the wrist

**semilunar valve** [sem-ee-LEW-nar valv] half-moon-shaped valve between the heart and the aorta that prevents blood flow from the aorta into the left ventricle during ventricular relaxation

**semimembranosus muscle** [sem-ee-mem-bruh-NOH-sus MUS-sel] one of three muscles of the posterior thigh that flexes the knee; extends and rotates the hip when contracted

**seminal vesicle** [SEM-ih-nal VES-ih-kal] structure of the testicle that secretes an alkaline fluid into the ejaculatory duct

**seminiferous tubules** [SEM-ih-NIF-er-us TOO-byoolz] channels or long tubules located in the testes

**semitendinosus muscle** [SEM-ee-ten-di-NOH-sus MUS-sel] one of three muscles of the posterior thigh that has a thick tendon attached at the ischium and ends at the medial condyle of the tibia; functions to flex the knee, and extend and rotate the hip

**senile plaques** [SEE-nyl plaks] clinical finding, associated with Alzheimer's disease, of abnormal amyloid deposits in brain tissue that disrupt brain function

**sensorineural hearing loss** [SEN-soh-ree-NYOOR-al HEER-ing loss] decreased ability to perceive sound due to damage to the hair cells in the cochlea

**sensory nerve** [SEN-sor-ee nerv] neurological tissue that transmits experiences of sound, light, position, pressure, heat, and cold to the brain

**sensory neuron** [SEN-sor-ee NYOO-ron] nerves that transmit information back to the central nervous system from the periphery; also known as afferent neuron

**sepsis** [SEP-sis] an inflammatory response to infection characterized by fever, increased heart and respiratory rates, and decreased blood pressure

**septicemia** [SEP-tih-SEE-mee-ah] presence of bacterial infection in the blood

**septotomy** [SEPT-ot-oh-mee] incision into the septum of any dividing structure, especially the nasal septum

**septum** [SEP-tum] tissue that divides a cavity or space into two parts

**sequela** [see-KWEL-ah] a condition resulting from a previous disease or disorder; plural is sequelae

**seroconversion** [SER-oh-kon-VER-shun] process where exposure to a pathogen causes a change from negative to a positive finding of antibodies for that pathogen; often observed with tuberculosis

**serotonin** [SER-oh-TOH-nin] a neurotransmitter in the central nervous system which stimulates smooth-muscle contraction in the intestinal tract

**serous** [SEER-us] a watery, serum-like fluid secreted by the serous membrane that is similar to clear liquid serum of the blood

**serum gastric test** [SEER-um GAS-trik test] laboratory test used to determine level of gastrin in blood serum

**serum lipase** [SEER-um LIP-ace] test measuring pancreatic enzyme levels of lipase in the blood

**sesamoid bone** [ses-ah-MOYD bohn] a small ovoid bone embedded in a tendon that lies over a joint and does not articulate with another bone; for example, the patella

**sessile polyp** [ses-SIL POL-ip] pendulous soft tissue arising from a mucus membrane with a broad base attachment

**sexually transmitted disease** [SEKS-yoo-al-ee tranz-MIT-tid dis-EEZ] infectious conditions spread by sexual contact, including syphilis, *Chlamydia*, AIDS, gonorrhea, and others

**shin splints** [SHIN splintz] pain in the anterior tibial region; disorder associated with inflammation and microtears of the tibial periosteum and related extensor muscles due to tremendous muscle stress caused by running on hard surfaces

**shingles** [SHING-lz] painful raised lesions along nerve roots

**short bowel syndrome** [short BOW-el SIN-drom] decreased ability to digest and absorb foods due to reduced length of intestine; this may be the result of congenital defects, infection, or extensive necrotizing enterocolitis

**sialolith** [sigh-AL-oh-lith] stone formed by the body

**sialolithiasis** [sigh-AL-oh-lith-AYE-sis] a stone formed in the salivary gland which becomes lodged in the duct, blocking the flow of saliva and resulting in painful swelling of the salivary gland, face, or mouth

**sialorrhea** [sy-ah-loh-REE-ah] excess production of saliva, or increased retention of saliva in the mouth, due to difficulty swallowing

**siccant** [SIK-ant] agent that removes moisture or promotes dryness of tissue or a body surface

**sickle-cell anemia** [SIK-kul-SEL ah-NEE-mee-ah] hereditary hemoglobinopathy, with partial or complete replacement of normal hemoglobin with abnormal hemoglobin

**sigmoid colon** [SIG-moyd KO-lon] an S-shaped section of bowel preceded by the descending colon, terminating at the anus

**sigmoidoscope** [SIG-moyd-oh-SKOHP] instrument used to visualize the sigmoid colon

**silicosis** [sil-ih-KOH-sis] pneumoconiosis caused by inhalation of silica dust, often seen in quarry or stone masons who experience occupational exposure

**single-photon emission computed tomography** [sing-al-FOH-ton ee-MIS-shun kom-PYOO-ted toh-MOG-rah-fee] a nuclear imaging study of organ(s) following the injection of a radioactive tracer

**sinoatrial node** [sigh-no-AYE-tree-al nohd] a dense network of fibers at the junction of the superior vena cava and the right atrium, where electrical impulses originate

**sinus** [SY-nus] a cavity or space within a structure

**sinus tachycardia** [SY-nus tak-ee-KAR-dee-ah] heart rate with normal rhythm but elevated rate above 100 beats per minute

**sinusotomy** [sy-nus-AW-toh-mee] surgical incision into a sinus

**-sis** [sis] *suffix*; condition or state

**Sjögren syndrome** [SHOE-greyn SIN-drom] autoimmune disease marked by dry skin, dry nasal membranes, and multiple areas of arthritis

**skeletal traction** [SKEL-eh-tal TRAK-shun] use of pins, wires, or tongs inserted into the bone during surgery to align the bone fragments

**skin traction** [skin TRAK-shun] use of elastic wraps, straps, halters, or skin adhesives connected to a pulley and weights, to align a body part following surgery or a fracture

**sleep apnea** [sleep AP-nee-uh] cessation of breathing during sleep that causes awakening and is characterized by daytime sleepiness

**slit-lamp examination** [SLIT-lamp ex-am-in-AY-shun] diagnostic procedure to detect abnormalities of the cornea, anterior chamber, iris, or lens using a low-power microscope (biomicroscope) for magnification with a high-intensity light

**socket** [SOH-kit] a hollow joint or acetabulum

**soleus muscle** [SOH-lee-us MUS-sel] muscle of the foot that causes plantar flexion when contracted

**soma** [SOH-muh] all cells in the body except bacteria

**somatization** [so-mah-ti-ZAY-shun] process of expressing emotional distress by physical complaints

**somatostatin** [SOH-mah-to-STAT-in] a peptide responsible for the regulation and inhibition of hormones by various neuroendocrine cells in the brain and gastrointestinal tract

**-some** [sohm] *suffix;* body

**somnolent** [SOM-no-lent] prolonged drowsiness, sedation, or sleepiness, often the result of disease or medications

**-spasm** [spa-zim] *suffix;* sudden, involuntary contraction

**spastic athetosis** [SPAZ-tik ath-eh-TOH-sis] constant involuntary writhing motions that are most often due to an extrapyramidal lesion

**spastic paralysis** [spaz-TIK pa-RAL-ih-sis] stiff and awkward muscle control caused by a central nervous system disorder

**specific gravity** [spe-SIF-ik GRAV-ih-tee] measure of the density of the urine compared to that of water

**spermatic** [sper-MAT-ik] pertaining to spermatozoon

**spermatogenesis** [SPER-mah-toh-JEN-eh-sis] the process of forming mature spermatozoa

**spermatozoa** [SPER-mah-tah-ZOH-ah] a mature sperm cell

**sphincter** [SFINGK-ter] a muscle that encircles a duct or tube in such a manner that constriction closes the orifice or lumen

**sphincter of Oddi** [SFINK-ter uv OD-ee] a circular muscle in the common bile duct that opens to permit passage of bile and pancreatic secretions into the duodenum

**sphygmomanometer** [sfing-moh-man-OM-et-ur] instrument used to measure blood pressure in millimeters of mercury; abbreviated mm Hg

**sphygmus** [SFIG-mus] pulse or pulsating quality

**spica hip cast** [SPY-kah hip kast] a rigid cast of the lower torso extending to one or both of the legs; used for femoral fractures

**spina bifida** [SPYE-nah BIF-ih-duh] a congenital defect resulting in incomplete closure of the vertebral column, usually in the lumbosacral region

**spina bifida cystica** [SPYE-nah BIF-ih-duh SIS-ti-kuh] the most severe type of spina bifida, characterized by increased intracranial pressure, meningocele, hydrocephalus, paraplegia, and the inability to control urinary bladder or rectum

**spina bifida occulta** [SPYE-nah BIF-ih-duh oh-KULT-ah] incomplete fusion of the vertebral posterior arch without protrusion as the lesion is covered by skin and generally evident only on x-ray evaluation

**spinal** [SPY-nal] pertaining to the backbone or vertebrae

**spinal cord** [SPY-nal kord] major nervous tissue originating at the base of the skull and terminating at the area between the first and third lumbar vertebra

**spinal nerves** [SPY-nal nervs] the 31 paired nerves originating from the spinal cord and containing afferent and efferent fibers to send and receive nervous impulses

**spine** [SPYN] vertical column of bones composed of 24 individual vertebrae plus the sacrum and coccyx

**spiral fracture** [SPY-ral FRAK-shur] this fracture occurs when a bone is broken because of a twisting force

**spleen** [SPLEEN] a nonvital, highly vascular organ involved with lymphocyte production; located in the left hypochondriac region

**splenectomy** [spleen-NEK-toh-mee] surgical removal of the spleen when it has ruptured due to trauma

**splenic vein** [SPLEN-ik vayn] vascular structure that carries deoxygenated blood away from the spleen to the portal vein

**splenius capitis muscle** [SPLEE-nee-us KAP-ih-tis MUS-sel] a muscle of the dorsal surface of the head that, when contracted, pulls the head into an upright position

**splenocele** [SPLEE-noh-seel] herniation of the spleen

**splenomegaly** [SPLEN-oh-MEG-ah-lee] enlargement of the spleen, detectable with palpation of the abdomen; possible causes are mononucleosis, Hodgkin's disease, hemolytic anemia, polycythemia vera, and leukemia

**splenorrhaphy** [splee-NOR-ah-fee] profuse bleeding from the spleen due to laceration or rupture

**spondylolisthesis** [SPAWN-dih-LOH-lis-THEE-sis] degenerative condition of the spine in which one vertebra moves anteriorly due to degeneration of the intervertebral disc; often due to traumatic injury or compression fracture of the vertebra from osteoporosis

**spontaneous fracture** [spawn-TAY-nee-us FRAK-shur] breakage of a bone resulting from an underlying disease such as osteoporosis

**sprain** [SPRAYN] overstretching or tearing of a ligament; treated by rest, immobilization, or surgery to repair the ligament

**sputum** [SPEW-tum] fluid or semifluid material discharged from the mouth, air passages, and throat

**squamous cell carcinoma** [SKWAY-mus sell kahr-si-NOH-muh] cancer that develops in the epidermis

**ST interval** [ess-tee IN-ter-val] segment of an electrocardiogram tracing that indicates time between ventricular contractions

**-stalsis** [stal-sis] *suffix*; contraction

**staphylococcus** [STAF-ih-loh-KOK-kus] a class of bacterium that has a characteristic clumping quality similar to a cluster of grapes; causes pyrogenic infections

**Starling's law of the heart** [STAR-lingz law uv the HART] the force of heart contraction is determined by the length of cardiac heart muscle fibers, and therefore, the further they stretch during diastole, the greater the force of the heartbeat

**-stasis** [stay-sis] *suffix*; standstill, or unmoving

**stasis dermatitis** [STAY-sis der-mah-TY-tis] inflammation of and increased pigmentation and thickening of the skin of the lower extremities due to decreased venous return

**statins** [STA-tinz] a pharmacological class of agents that reduce low-density lipids (LDL)

**status asthmaticus** [STA-tus az-MAT-ih-kus] a prolonged, extremely severe, life-threatening asthma attack

**steatoma** [stee-ah-TOH-mah] lipoma, fatty tumor

**steatorrhea** [stee-AT-oh-REE-uh] greasy, frothy, foul-smelling stools that contain undigested fats

**-stenosis** [sten-oh-sis] *suffix*; narrowed or constricted

**stereocilia** [ster-ee-oh-SIL-ee-ah] hair cells located in the inner ear; the hairs are involved with balance and equilibrium

**stereognosis** [ster-ee-og-NOH-sis] mental ability to perceive the form and nature of objects by touch; tested as part of neurological assessment

**stereoscopic vision** [ster-ee-oh-SKOP-ik VIH-zhun] three-dimensional vision with depth perception

**sternal** [STER-nal] pertaining to the breastbone

**sternal retraction** [STER-nal re-TRAK-shun] inward movement of the breastbone associated with respiratory distress syndrome

**sternocleidomastoid muscle** [STER-noh-klye-doh-MAS-toyd MUS-sel] muscle that flexes the neck in a forward motion

**sternohyoid muscle** [ster-noh-HIGH-oyd MUS-sel] a muscle that extends from the medial aspect of the clavicle and sternum to the hyoid bone of the neck and depresses the hyoid bone and larynx when contracted

**sternum** [STER-num] long, narrow, flat bone of the medial chest; breastbone

**Stevens-Johnson syndrome** [STEE-venz-JON-son SIN-drom] a systemic skin disorder with fever and blistering lesions of the skin and of all mucous membranes, including the mouth and conjunctivae, resulting in dehydration, infection, sepsis, and possibly death

**stimulation** [STIM-yoo-LAY-shun] the irritating or arousing of muscles, nerves, or other sensory organs

**stockinet** [stok-in-ET] a tubular elastic mesh device that holds dressings in place on the trunk, head, and extremities

**stoma** [STOH-mah] an artificially created opening on the surface of the body, such as a colostomy or tracheostomy

**stomach** [STUM-ak] a muscular structure that is situated between the esophagus and duodenum, and secretes hydrochloric acid and other digestive juices

**stomatitis** [STO-mah-TY-tis] inflammation of the oral mucosa which can be caused by poorly fitting dentures that rub the gums

**-stomy** [stohm-ee] *suffix*; creation of an artificial opening

**strabismus** [strah-BIZ-mus] disorder of the eye alignment where one eye deviates from the point of focus

**strangulated hernia** [STRANG-yoo-lay-ted HUR-nee-ah] abnormal protrusion of the intestine through the abdominal wall, obstructing blood flow and fecal movement

**stratum** [STRAY-tum] a thin layer of tissue having uniform thickness

**strawberry hemangioma** [STRAW-ber-ee he-man-jee-OH-muh] type of birthmark characterized by raised vascular nevus, commonly observed on the face or neck

**stress fracture** [STRESS FRAK-shur] fine-line disruption of bone integrity due to repetitive microtrauma

**stressor** [STRES-or] negative and positive life events

**stria** [STRY-uh] narrow marking band on skin; stretch marks

**striated muscle** [STRY-aye-ted MUS-sel] skeletal and cardiac muscles showing bands of color when examined under the microscope

**stricture** [STRIK-chur] constriction or narrowing of a lumen, duct, or organ such as the urethra, ureter, or esophagus

**stridor, respiratory** [STRY-dor, RES-pih-ra-tor-ee] an abnormally high-pitched sound during inspiration due to the constriction or narrowing of the larynx or trachea

**strumectomy** [stru-MEK-toh-mee] surgical excision of a portion or all of a tumor on the thyroid gland

**Stryker frame** [STRY-ker fraym] a structure that holds the patient on a bed; it can be rotated into different positions while keeping the patient's body from moving

**sub-** [sub] *prefix*; under or below

**subarachnoid space** [sub-ah-RAK-ah-noyd spays] the cerebrospinal fluid-filled area between the pia mater and the arachnoid surfaces of the brain

**subclavian artery** [sub-KLAY-vee-an AR-ter-ee] blood vessel that supplies oxygenated blood to the brain and face; palpable pulsation is called the subclavian pulse

**subclavian vein** [sub-KLAY-vee-an vayn] a large blood vessel that drains in the arm, joining with the internal jugular vein

**subclinical** [sub-KLIN-ih-kal] having mild or subtle indications of a disorder

**subcutaneous** [sub-kew-TAY-nee-us] connective tissue skin layer; hypodermis

**subdural** [sub-DUR-ahl] space between the dura mater and arachnoid matter of the brain

**sublingual (SL)** [sub-LIN-gwal] pertaining to the oral mucosal surface immediately under the tongue; often used as a delivery modality for medications in which the medication is allowed to dissolve under the tongue

**sublingual glands** [sub-LIN-gwal glandz] lymph nodules that drain the region of the throat and tonsils

**subluxation** [sub-luk-SAY-shun] incomplete dislocation where the articular surfaces are out of normal alignment but still in contact with each other

**submandibular** [sub-man-DIB-yoo-lar] pertaining to the area under the lower jaw

**submandibular nodes** [sub-man-DIB-yoo-lar nohdz] lymphatic tissue immediately beneath the lower jaw

**submandibularitis** [sub-man-DIB-yoo-lar-EYE-tis] inflammation of the lymph nodes below the lower jaw due to bacterial infection; commonly associated with mumps

**submental lymph nodes** [sub-MEN-tal LYMF nohdz] lymph nodes located under the chin that drain and circulate lymph from the head and throat region

**subscapularis muscle** [sub-SKAP-yoo-lahr-is MUS-sel] muscle that medially rotates the shoulder

**subtalar joint** [sub-TAY-lar joynt] articular surface between the talus and calcaneus bones of the foot

**subtendinous iliac bursa** [sub-TEN-dih-nus ILL-ee-ak BUR-sah] the sheath covering at the point of attachment for the iliopsoas muscle to the lesser trochanter of the femoral head

**sucrase** [SOO-krays] enzyme secreted by the small intestine to break sucrose into glucose

**sudoresis** [sue-doh-REE-sis] profuse sweating or perspiration

**sudoriferous glands** [sue-doh-RIF-er-us glandz] structures that produce sweat

**suffocative goiter** [SUF-oh-kay-tiv GOY-ter] enlargement of the thyroid gland that presses on the upper airway, producing respiratory stridor

**suggillation** [sug-ji-LAY-shun] bleeding under the skin; bruising

**suicidal ideation** [soo-ih-SY-dal EYE-dee-aye-shun] to entertain thoughts or make plans to end one's own life

**sundowning** [SUN-dow-ning] increased level of confusion, restlessness, and confusion in the late afternoon and evening hours in patients with dementia

**super-** [sue-per] *prefix*; above, high, or excessive

**superficial** [SUE-per-FISH-al] near the surface; shallow, not deep or penetrating

**superior** [soo-PEER-ee-or] situated above another structure; of higher quality

**superior hepatic vein** [soo-PEER-ee-or he-PAH-tik vayn] major blood vessel that moves blood away from the liver and intestinal tract

**superior oblique muscle** [soo-PEER-ee-or ob-LEEK MUS-sel] muscle that turns the eye upward and toward the midline of the visual field

**superior rectus muscle** [soo-PEER-ee-or REK-tus MUS-sel] muscle that turns the eye upward

**superior vena cava** [soo-PEER-ee-or VEE-na KAY-vah] large vessel that returns blood from the head, neck, and upper limbs, terminating at the right atrium

**supinator muscle** [SOO-pi-nay-tur MUS-sel] muscle that turns the forearm in a palm down position

**supine** [SOO-pyne] positioning of a patient lying on the back with the palms facing up

**suppository** [suh-PAWS-ih-tor-ee] a formed, bullet-shaped capsule that contains a drug for administration of medication by melting in the rectum where it is absorbed

**supra-** [sue-prah] *prefix*; above or excessive

**supra spinatus muscle** [SOO-prah spye-NAY-tus MUS-sel] muscle that abducts the shoulder

**suprapubic catheter** [sue-prah-PEW-bik KATH-eh-ter] insertion of a catheter into the bladder above the symphysis pubis bone using a surgical incision

**suprapubic prostatectomy** [soo-prah-PYOO-bik praws-tah-TEK-toh-mee] excision of the prostate gland by a superior approach above the symphysis pubis to avoid nerves to the penis

**suprarenal glands** [sue-pra-REE-nal glanz] an excretory structure that produces epinephrine, norepinephrine, and cortisone; also regulates carbohydrate metabolism, salt, and water balance

**supraventricular tachycardia** [SOO-prah-ven-TRIK-yoo-lar TAK-ee-KAR-dee-uh] common pathologic tachycardia characterized by abrupt onset of a rapid, regular heart rate, often too fast to count

**surfactant** [sur-FAK-tant] agent that lowers the surface tension of a liquid, such as mucous in the upper airway

**suspensory ligaments** [suh-SPENS-or-ee LIG-ah-mentz] fibrous tissue that serves the purpose of holding structures, such as the ovary and uterus, in anatomical position

**Swan-Ganz catheter** [swan-ganz KATH-eh-ter] a flexible catheter inserted into the pulmonary artery of patients in shock; used for hemodynamic monitoring

**sym-** [sim] *prefix;* with or together

**sympathetic ganglion** [sym-pah-THEH-tik GANG-lee-on] a collection of nerve cells that are attached to efferent fibers that originate from visceral motor neurons in the thoracic and upper lumbar spine

**symphysis pubis** [SIM-fi-sis PEW-bis] the fibrocartilaginous union of the pubic bones

**symptom** [SIMP-tom] a change in health experienced by a patient

**symptomology** [SIMP-tom-AWL-oh-jee] clinical representation of signs and symptoms associated with a disease

**syn-** [sin] *prefix;* with or together

**synapse** [SIN-aps] communicating region between neurons

**synaptic cleft** [syn-AP-tik kleft] a small, fluid-filled space between two neurons where neurotransmitters are released

**synaptic terminal** [syn-AP-tik TER-mih-nal] the end portion of an axon that receives the nerve impulse

**synaptic vesicle** [syn-AP-tik VES-ih-kl] a small, saclike structure at the end of the synapse that contains neurotransmitters

**synchia** [syn-KEE-ah] adhesion of tissues, particularly the iris, lens, and cornea

**synchondrosis** [sin-kon-DROH-sis] joint in which the surfaces are connected by a cartilage plate

**syncope** [SING-koh-pee] loss of consciousness due to inadequate oxygen to the brain

**syndactyly** [sin-DAK-tih-lee] congenital condition in which soft tissues of fingers or toes are joined

**syndesmosis** [syn-dez-MOH-sis] articulation in which the bones are held together by fibrous connective tissue

**syndesmotomy** [syn-des-MOT-oh-mee] surgical incision of ligaments

**syndrome** [SIN-drom] signs and symptoms of a particular disease

**synechotomy** [syn-ek-OT-oh-mee] surgical incision of an adhesion

**synechtenterotomy** [syn-EK-ten-ter-OT-oh-mee] surgical excision of adhesions of the intestine

**syphilis** [SIF-ih-lis] multiphase, sexually transmitted disease caused by infection with the organism *Treponema pallidum*

**syrigmus** [sir-IG-mus] subjective report of ringing or hissing sounds in the ears

**systematic desensitization** [sis-teh-MAT-ik dee-SEN-sih-tih-ZAY-shun] a technique in which a patient imagines multiple scenarios of progressively greater anxiety while utilizing relaxation techniques until they no longer cause anxiety; used as an adjunct to pharmacological therapies in treating severe anxiety

**systemic** [SIS-tem-ik] relating to the whole body

**systemic lupus erythematosus (SLE)** [sis-TEM-ik LOU-pus eh-rith-mah-TOH-sis] a chronic autoimmune inflammatory disease with characteristic facial "butterfly rash," involving hematologic, cardiac, pulmonary, and renal systems

**systole** [SIS-toh-lee] contraction of the heart muscle

**systolic blood pressure** [sis-TOL-ik BLUD presh-ur] arterial blood pressure during ventricular contraction

# T

**T wave** [TEE wayv] section of the electrocardiogram (ECG) showing ventricular repolarization

**tachy-** [tak-ee] *prefix*; swift or rapid

**tachycardia** [tak-ee-KAHR-dee-ah] rapid heart rate in excess of 100 beats per minute

**tachypnea** [tak-ip-NEE-uh] rapid respiratory rate

**tactile stimulation** [TAK-tile stim-yoo-LAY-shun] invoking a neurological response by touching

**talipes equinovarus** [TAY-lih-peez ee-KWY-noh-VAR-us] congenital deformity of one or both feet in which the foot is pulled downward and laterally; the heel never rests on the floor, causing the patient to walk on the toes; most common type of clubfoot

**talus** [TAY-lus] the first tarsal bone and the largest of the bones of the ankle, which articulates with the tibia and fibula

**tardive dyskinesia** [TAR-dive DIS-kih-NEE-zee-ah] a complication of treatment with antipsychotic medications that produces abnormal, involuntary, repetitive movements of the face (grimacing, lip smacking, eye blinking, tongue movements) and can also include movements of the arms and legs

**Tarlov cysts** [TAHR-lov sistz] perineural cysts located in the proximal radicles of the lower spinal cord which produce symptoms of nerve pain

**tarsal** [TAR-sol] pertaining to the seven individual bones that make up the ankle

**T-cells** [TEE-sells] thymus-derived lymphocytes that recognize and kill cancerous cells and cells infected with viruses or identified as foreign tissue

**temporal artery** [tem-POR-al AR-ter-ee] blood vessel that brings oxygenated blood to the brain

**temporal bone** [tem-POR-al bohn] segment of the cranium located on the sides of the head, anterior to the ears

**temporal foramen** [TEM-poh-ral FOR-aye-men] a small opening in the cranium for the ear canal

**temporal lobe** [tem-POR-al lohb] lateral segments of the cerebrum under the temporal bone

**temporalis muscle** [tem-poh-RAL-is MUS-sel] smooth muscle of the lateral surface of the face

**temporomandibular joint syndrome** [TEM-poh-roh-man-DIB-yoo-lar JOYNT SIN-drom] dysfunction of the temporomandibular joint with clicking, pain, muscle spasm, and difficulty opening the jaw; caused by chewing on only one side of the mouth, clenching or grinding the teeth during sleep, or misalignment of the teeth

**tendolysis** [ten-DOL-eye-is] releasing a tendon from adhesions

**tendons** [TEN-dunz] fibrous bands or cords that attach muscle to bone or muscle to other body parts

**tendoplasty** [TEN-do-plas-tee] surgical repair of a tendon to restore functionality

**tenotomy** [teh-NOT-oh-mee] surgical resection of a tendon

**tensor fasciae latae muscle** [TEN-sor FASH-ee-aye LAY-tah MUS-sel] muscle of the hip that extends the hip when contracted

**teratogenic** [ter-ah-toh-JEN-ik] affecting the development of a fetus, as in transmitting or causing malformation

**teres major muscle** [TEER-eez MAY-jor MUS-sel] muscle that extends and medially rotates shoulder

**teres minor muscle** [TEER-eez MY-nohr MUS-sel] muscle that rotates the arm laterally

**terminal** [TER-mih-nal] pertaining to the end boundary, especially a disease from which a patient cannot recover or that is likely to cause death

**testicle** [TES-tih-kul] male gonad which functions to produce sperm and testosterone; singular form of testes

**testosterone** [tes-TAWS-ter-rohn] sex hormone responsible for masculine characteristics: maturation of sexual organs, spermatogenesis, sex drive, erectile capabilities, facial hair, and pronounced musculature

**tetanus** [TET-ah-nus] infection with the bacillus *Clostridium tetani* in deep puncture wounds; characterized by gross muscular rigidity, severe muscle spasms, respiratory failure, and death

**tetany** [TET-ah-nee] painful intermittent muscle spasms frequently associated with calcium imbalance

**tetra-** [tet-rah] *prefix*; four

**tetraiodothyronine** [tet-rah-eye-oh-doh-THIGH-roh-nine] thyroid hormone

**tetralogy of Fallot** [te-TRAL-oh-jee uv fahl-OH] four congenital heart defects appearing together

**tetranopsia** [tet-rah-NOP-see-ah] loss of one-fourth of the visual field

**tetraparesis** [tet-rah-PAR-ee-sis] muscular weakness in all four extremities

**thalamus** [THAL-ah-mus] gray matter on either side of the third ventricle of the brain that acts as a relay station for impulses from the sensory nerves and sends them to specific cortical areas of the brain

**thallium** [THAL-ee-um] assessment of coronary artery disease by use of a radioactive isotope of thallium administered by an intravenous drip, followed by a physical stress test; the isotope collects in areas of decreased circulation and can be visualized on the scanner

**thanatophobia** [THAN-ah-toh-FOH-bee-ah] fear of death

**therapy vest** [THER-ah-pee vest] a vestlike garment that vibrates, shaking the chest wall in efforts to break up mucus from lung fields for expectoration or suctioning

**thermoreceptor** [ther-moh-ree-SEP-tor] sensory sites that are stimulated by the rise in temperature

**thermoregulation** [THER-moh-reg-yoo-LAY-shun] efforts by the hypothalamus to maintain body temperature by heat production and heat loss

**theta waves** [THAY-tah wayvz] brain waves seen on electroencephalography; most often found in children, but may occur in adults under emotional stress

**thimerosal** [thigh-MER-oh-sal] a mercury compound used to preserve pharmacological agents and vaccines

**third-degree burn** [third-deh-GREE burn] destruction of the full thickness of the skin and underlying structures due to chemical or thermal exposure

**thoracentesis** [THOR-ah-sen-TEE-sis] removal of fluid from the thoracic cavity, usually due to cancer or pneumonia

**thoracic** [thoh-RAS-ik] pertaining to the chest

**thoracic lymph duct** [thoh-RAS-ik LIMF dukt] the common trunk of all lymphatic vessels in the body except those from the right neck and head area

**thoracic outlet compression syndrome** [thoh-RAS-ik OUT-let kom-PRESH-un SIN-drom] compression of nerves and/or blood vessels of the neck due to entrapment between the pectoralis minor and adjacent muscles, resulting in decreased sensation and blood supply to the upper extremities

**thoracic spine** [thoh-RAS-ik SPYN] the region of the 12 bony segments of the spinal column of the upper back, designated T1 to T12

**thoracic vertebrae** [thoh-RAS-ik VER-teh-bray] the 12 discs of the spinal column that connect the ribs, forming the posterior wall of the thorax

**thoracocentesis** [thor-ah-koh-sen-TEE-sis] removal of fluid from the chest cavity using a surgical puncture, usually a large-bore needle

**thoracometer** [tho-rah-KOM-eh-ter] medical device used to measure the expansion of the chest during inspiration

**thoracoplasty** [THOR-ah-koh-plas-tee] surgical removal of portions of the ribs to collapse diseased portions of the lung in efforts to treat pulmonary tuberculosis and empyema

**thoracotomy** [thor-ah-KOT-oh-mee] surgical incision of the chest wall, usually performed laterally between the ribs

**thorax** [THOR-aks] portion of the body below the base of the neck and above the diaphragm; further divided into the anterior, posterior, and axillary surfaces

**thromboangiitis obliterans** [throm-boh-an-jee-EYE-tis uh-BLIT-ur-anz] inflammation and decreased blood flow in the peripheral arteries and veins of the extremities caused by long-term tobacco use; also known as Buerger disease

**thrombocytopenia** [THRAWM-boh-sy-toh-PEE-nee-ah] deficiency of thrombocytes due to action or chemicals or drugs that damage stem cells in the bone marrow; also occurs when leukemia cells take over and crowd the stem cells that produce thrombocytes

**thrombocytosis** [throm-boh-sy-TOH-sis] mildly increased number of platelets in circulation

**thrombolytic** [throm-boh-LIT-ik] dissolution of blood clots by breaking down the fibrin strands

**thrombophlebitis** [throm-boh-fleb-EYE-tis] vein inflammation and thrombus (clot) formation

**thrombosis** [throm-BOH-sis] formation or presence of a clot in a blood vessel

**thymectomy** [thigh-MEK-toh-mee] surgical removal of the thymus due to a tumor or myasthenia gravis

**-thymia** [thigh-mee-uh] *suffix*; state of mind

**thymoma** [thigh-MOH-mah] a tumor of the thymus which is usually benign

**thymosins** [THIGH-moh-sins] an endocrine gland that produces lymphocytes and regulates the immune system; located posterior to the sternum between the lungs

**thymus** [THIGH-mus] a lymph organ located in the anterosuperior mediastinum

**thyroid** [THIGH-roid] the gland that secretes thyroid hormones

**thyroid cancer** [THIGH-royd KAN-ser] malignant neoplasm of the thyroid gland; there are four types: papillary, follicular, medullary, and undifferentiated; treatment has a very high success rate

**thyroid cartilage** [THIGH-royd KAR-tih-laj] V-shaped structure surrounding the larynx that forms a subcutaneous projection; commonly referred to as the "Adam's apple"

**thyroid scan** [THIGH-royd skan] diagnostic nuclear scan in which a radioactive substance is injected and uptake by the thyroid gland is measured using a gamma camera

**thyroid stimulating hormone (TSH)** [THIGH-royd STIM-yoo-lay-ting HOR-mohn] substance secreted by the pituitary gland that triggers the thyroid gland to produce thyroxine and triiodothyronine

**thyroidectomy** [thigh-royd-EK-toh-mee] partial or complete surgical removal of the thyroid gland

**thyrotoxic** [THIGH-roh-TOK-sik] crisis exacerbation of the symptoms of hyperthyroidism; thyroid storm

**thyrotoxicosis** [thigh-roh-tok-si-KOH-sis] condition of excessive thyroid hormone

**thyroxine (T₄)** [THIGH-roks-in] one of the hormones secreted by the thyroid gland responsible for metabolic rate and processing of all types of food and protein synthesis in bodily tissues

**tibia** [TIB-ee-ah] small bone of the anterior surface of the lower leg

**tibialis anterior muscle** [tib-ee-AH-lis an-TEER-ee-or MUS-sel] muscle of the anterior lower leg that flexes the foot and ankle when contracted

**tibialis muscle** [tib-ee-AL-is MUS-sel] acts to produce anterior inversion of the foot

**tibiofemoral joint** [tib-ee-oh-FEM-uh-rul JOYNT] the articular surface of the tibia and femur; knee joint

**-tic** [tik] *suffix*; pertaining to

**tidal volume (TV)** [TYE-dal VOL-yoom] volume of air moved in or out of the lungs during normal breathing

**tinea** [TIN-ee-uh] lesions of dermatophytoses which may present in the feet (pedi), nails (unguium), groin area (cruris), or any superficial skin surface (versicolor)

**Tinel's test** [tih-NELZ test] assessment for carpal tunnel syndrome where the patient's arms are tapped with a reflex hammer; positive report of "pins and needles" sensation is diagnostic for carpal tunnel syndrome

**tinnitus** [tin-EYE-tus] ringing sensation in the ear

**-tion** [shun] *suffix*; condition or state

**tissue plasminogen activator** [TISH-yoo plaz-MIN-oh-jen AK-tih-vay-tor] an enzymatic substance that acts to dissolve blood clots; used therapeutically following myocardial infarction to restore blood supply to heart muscle

**titer** [TY-ter] a standardized measurement of the concentration of a substance in a solution; often used to measure the presence of immune response to vaccinations

**-tocia** [toh-see-ah] *suffix*; labor; to give birth

**tocolysis** [toh-koh-LYE-sis] inhibition or prevention of uterine contractions in efforts to delay delivery of a fetus

**tolerance** [TAWL-er-ans] progressive decrease in therapeutic effect of a drug or therapy

**-tome** [tohm] *suffix*; instrument used for a particular purpose

**tomography** [toh-MOG-rah-fee] procedure of making a radiographic image of a selected physical plane for diagnostic purposes

**-tomy** [toh-mee] *suffix*; incision or cut

**tongue** [TUNG] muscular organ of the mouth involved with taste and management of oral secretions

**tonic** [TAWN-ik] continuous muscular contraction; often used to describe seizure activity

**tonic-clonic movements** [TAWN-ik-KLAWN-ik MOOV-mentz] stiffening and jerking of all major motor muscle groups; previously known as grand-mal seizure

**tonometry** [toh-NAWM-eh-tree] diagnostic procedure to detect increased intraocular pressure indicative of glaucoma

**tonsillectomy** [ton-sih-LEK-toh-mee] surgical excision of the tonsils

**tonsillitis** [TAWN-sih-LY-tis] acute or chronic bacterial infection of the palatine tonsils and pharynx producing difficulty swallowing, edema and hypertrophy of tonsillar crypts, and blockage of the eustachian tubes

**tonsils** [TAWN-silz] lymphatic tissue located at the back of the throat that detect and respond to infection of the throat

**torpid** [TOR-pid] sluggish movements and/or slowed reactions due to neurological pathology such as drug side effects, anoxia, or brain trauma; also, sluggish or delayed responses associated with Parkinson's disease

**Tourette's syndrome** [TOOR-etz SIN-drom] frequent, spontaneous, involuntary body-movement tics (eye blinking, throat clearing, arm thrusting) and vocal tics (grunts, barks), or comments that are socially inappropriate, vulgar, or obscene

**torticollis** [tor-tih-KOL-is] stiff, spasmodic neck typically producing lateral flexion of the muscles of the cervical spine

**tortuous** [TOR-choo-us] twisted, sinuous, wavy; as seen in varicose veins

**total anomalous pulmonary venous return** [TOH-tal ah-NOM-ah-lus PUHL-moh-nair-ee VEE-nus ree-TURN] a congenital heart defect in which the pulmonary veins empty into the right atrium or veins leading to the right atrium

**total lung capacity (TLC)** [TOE-tal lung ka-PAS-ih-tee] volume of air that the lungs can hold, defined as the vital capacity combined with the residual volume; average value = 6,000 cc

**toxigenicity** [toks-ih-jen-IS-ih-tee] relative potency of a poison-producing organism

**trabecular meshwork** [trah-BEK-yoo-lar MESH-wurk] area of interlacing fibers in which the aqueous humor is filtered; located in the region where the edges of the iris and the cornea meet

**trabeculoplasty** [trah-BEK-yoo-loh-PLAS-tee] surgical procedure used to treat glaucoma, where an argon laser is used to create small holes in half of the trabecular meshwork to increase the flow of aqueous humor

**trachea** [TRAY-kee-ah] a round cartilaginous structure of the upper airway that extends from the larynx to the bronchiole tubes

**trachealis muscle** [tray-kee-AH-lis MUS-sel] a muscle of the throat that decreases the lumen of the tracheal rings when contracted

**trachelodynia** [tray-keh-loh-DIN-ee-uh] pain in the neck

**trachelokyphosis** [tray-keh-low-ky-FOH-sis] abnormal or excessive anterior curvature of the cervical neck

**tracheobronchial suction** [TRAY-kee-oh-BRON-kee-al SUK-shun] use of a cannula to remove mucus, pus, or aspirated material from the trachea and upper bronchus to improve air exchange

**tracheobronchial tree** [TRAY-ke-oh-BRONK-ee-al tree] the inverted treelike structure of the trachea, main stem bronchi, and bronchioles; also known as bronchial tree

**tracheomalacia** [TRAY-kee-oh-ma-LAY-sha] degeneration of elastic and connective tissues in the trachea

**tracheostenosis** [TRAY-kee-oh-sten-OH-sis] narrowing of the lumen of the trachea

**tracheostomy** [TRAY-kee-AWS-toh-mee] an incision into the trachea creating a permanent opening to allow for a patent or open airway

**traction** [TRAK-shun] the process of putting a limb, bone, or group of muscles under tension by means of weights and pulleys to align or immobilize the part to reduce muscle spasm or to relieve pressure

**tragus** [TRAY-gus] the small frontal portion of ear cartilage near the auditory canal

**tranquilizer** [TRAN-kwih-LYZ-er] a major class of drugs used to relieve anxiety and tension, ranging from benzodiazepines to neuroleptics

**trans-** [trahns] *prefix*; across or through

**transcatheter closure** [tranz-KATH-eh-ter KLOH-zur] repair of a septal defect using a septal occluder or Rashkind device during cardiac catheterization

**transcutaneous electrical nerve stimulation (TENS)** [TRANS-kyoo-TAY-nee-us ee-LEK-trik-al nerv stim-yoo-LAY-shun] application of mild electrical current to the skin over a painful region, providing pain relief by interfering with transmission of pain signals

**transdermal** [trans-DERM-al] administration or absorption of a drug through intact skin

**transesophageal echocardiography** [TRAS-eh-sof-uh-GEE-al ek-oh-kar-dee-OG-rah-fee] examination of the heart using an endoscope and sonographic transducer inserted in the esophagus directly behind the heart

**transferrin** [trans-FAIR-in] blood chemistry test to determine the total iron-binding capacity of the blood

**transfusion** [trans-FYOO-zhun] injection of solutions, blood, and/or chemotherapeutic agents into a vein for therapeutic purposes

**transient ischemic attack** [tran-SEE-ent is-KEE-mik ah-TAK] temporary interference with blood supply to the brain by small clots, causing no permanent brain damage

**transplantation** [TRANZS-plan-TAY-shun] implantation of a living body part, organ, or tissue graft from a donor

**transposition of the great arteries (TGA)** [tranz-poh-SIZH-shun uv the grayt AR-ter-eez] condition where the pulmonary artery is the outflow for left ventricle, and the aorta is the outflow for right ventricle; life-threatening at birth, and survival initially depends on open ducts of arteriosus and foramen ovale; this condition occurs in about 5 percent of children with congenital heart disease

**transsexualism** [tranz-SEK-shoo-ah-lizm] belief of an individual that he or she has been assigned (by anatomy, parents, or society) the wrong gender identity, and needs to change his or her outward appearance to the opposite sex in order to match what is already felt in the mind

**transurethral resection** [TRANS-yoo-REE-thral ree-SEK-shun] the surgical removal of a structure performed through the urethra

**transverse** [trans-VERS] a horizontal plane that divides the body into two sections: upper and lower

**transverse fracture** [trans-VERS FRAK-shur] a bone break that is perpendicular to the bone's long axis

**transversus abdominis muscle** [trans-VUR-sus ab-DOM-ih-nis MUS-sel] muscle that compresses the abdomen and aids in posture

**trapezium** [tra-PEE-zee-um] a four-sided bone of the wrist that articulates with the base of the thumb

**trapezius muscle** [trah-PEE-zee-us MUS-sel] a flat, triangular muscle of the posterior shoulder and neck that shrugs the shoulder when flexed

**tremor** [TREM-or] involuntary shaking of a body part due to pathological states such as Parkinson's disease or side effects of medications; some subtypes include intention, coarse, fine, and resting, often detected in the hands and upper body

**Trendelenburg position** [tren-DEL-en-berg po-SISH-un] placement of a patient lying flat in bed with the head lowered and the feet elevated to enhance blood flow to the brain and vital organs

**tri-** [try] *prefix*; three

**triceps** [TRY-seps] having three heads or subdivisions

**triceps brachii muscle** [TRY-seps BRAY-kee-eye MUS-sel] muscle on the dorsal surface of the humerus that extends the forearm when flexed

**trichomycosis** [trik-oh-migh-KOH-sis] fungal hair disease

**trichotillomania** [TRIK-oh-TIL-oh-MAY-nee-ah] repetitive pulling out of hair from the head

**tricuspid atresia** [try-KUS-pid ah-TREE-see-ah] congenital absence of the tricuspid valve of the heart

**tricuspid valve** [try-KUS-pid valv] a structure of the heart that allows blood to flow in one direction from the right atrium to the right ventricle

**trigeminal neuralgia** [trye-JEM-ih-nul new-RHAL-juh] pain in one or more branches of cranial nerve V

**trigeminy** [try-JEM-ih-nee] occurrence of events in groups of three, especially three rapid heartbeats

**triglyceride** [try-GLIS-er-yd] a simple fat molecule consisting of three molecules of fatty acids and glycerol; they combine with lipoproteins in the blood and are stored in body tissues as fat

**triiodothyronine (T3)** [tri-eye-oh-doh-THY-roh-neen] one of the hormones secreted by the thyroid gland

**-tripsy** [trip-see] *suffix*; to crush

**-trophy** [tro-fee] *suffix*; to nourish or develop

**troponin I** [TRO-po-nin wun] a highly sensitive and specific indicator of recent cardiac muscle damage

**trousseau sign** [true-SOH sighn] carpal tetany elicited when the brachial or forearm region is compressed due to hypocalcemia

**true ribs** [TRU ribz] the first seven pairs of curved bones that form the upper thoracic cage and are individually attached by cartilage to the sternum

**true vocal cords** [tru voh-KAL kordz] lower folds of the larynx that produce sound by vibrating as air moves out of the lungs

**truncus arteriosus** [TRUN-kus ar-tee-ree-OH-sis] heart malformation in which a single large vessel empties both ventricles, causing cyanosis to develop soon after birth with severe congestive heart failure, dyspnea, retractions, fatigue, polycythemia, clubbing, increased pulse pressure, bounding peripheral pulses, and cardiomegaly

**truss** [TRUHS] an externally applied device used to apply pressure to a hernia to prevent it from enlarging or protruding

**tubal ligation** [TU-bal lye-GAY-shun] female sterilization by surgical excision and closure of the fallopian tube so that conception cannot occur

**tubercles** [TOO-ber-klz] small lesions of inflammation associated with tuberculosis

**tuberculosis** [too-BER-kyoo-LOH-sis] a chronic granulomatous infection caused by an acid-fast bacillus, *Mycobacterium tuberculosis*

**tubule** [TOO-byool] a series of compartmentalized, small tubes that collect or transport substances in bodily organs

**tumescence** [tyoo-MES-ens] condition of being swollen or with edema

**tumor suppressor genes** [TOO-mor soo-PRES-sor jeenz] genetic material that controls the growth of cells, decreasing the effects of cancer-producing stimuli

**tunica** [TOO-ni-kah] fibro-elastic tissue that covers or coats tubular structures such as blood or lymph vessels

**tunica externa** [TOO-ni-kah ecks-TUR-nah] outermost layer of connective tissue covering an organ or structure that is not covered by a serosa

**tunica media** [TOO-ni-kah MEE-dee-ah] middle layer of the coating of a blood or lymph vessel; comprised of smooth muscle

**turbidimetry** [tur-bih-DIM-eh-tree] measurement of the relative cloudiness of a solution, such as urine, in which the amount of light able to pass through the substance is quantified by using a spectrophotometer

**turbinate** [TER-bin-ayt] coil-like structures, one on each side of the nasal septum, that act as barriers to divide and slow the passage of inhaled air so that it can pick up warmth and moisture

**turgor** [TUR-gur] normal skin tension

**Turner's syndrome** [TUR-nerz SIN-drom] a chromosomal anomaly occurring in approximately 1 in 3,000 births due to the absence of one X chromosome; characterized by webbing of neck skin, cardiovascular abnormalities, ovarian failure, shield-shaped chest, and underdevelopment of breast, uterus, and vagina

**tussis** [TUS-is] coughing

**tympani** [tym-PAN-ee] loud, high-pitched sounds similar to a drum, usually heard over an air-filled stomach

**tympanic membrane** [tym-PAN-ik MEM-brayn] a structure that is a thick but pliable tissue that registers sound and causes vibrations to be transmitted to the inner ear; also known as the eardrum

**tympanogram** [tim-PAN-oh-gram] a graphic record of the movement of the tympanic membrane in response to air-pressure changes in the external auditory canal

**tympanometry** [TIM-pah-NAWM-eh-tree] a hearing test that measures the ability of the tympanic membrane in the ear to move in response to air pressure (rather than sound)

**tympanoplasty** [tim-pah-no-PLAS-tee] surgical reconstruction of a ruptured tympanic membrane

**tympanotomy tubes** [tym-pan-AWT-oh-mee toobz] surgical insertion of small Teflon tubes in the tympanic membrane to equalize pressure, promote fluid drainage, and ventilate the middle ear

**Tzanck** [ZANK] a differential skin test using Giemsa stain with microscopic examination

# U

**-ula** [uhle-uh] *suffix*; small

**ulcer** [UL-sur] slow-healing sore on the surface of an organ or tissue resulting from tissue necrosis

**ulcerative colitis** [UL-ser-ah-tiv koh-LY-tis] an inflammatory disease of the ileum and colon with inflammation followed by areas of normal mucosa known as enteritis; the disease affects the colon and rectum; treatment may involve steroids and removal of affected segments of intestine

**ulcerative keratitis** [UL-ser-ah-tiv KER-ah-ty-tis] erosion of the cornea

**-ule** [uhle] *suffix*; small

**ulna** [UL-nah] forearm bone located along the little-finger side of the lower arm

**ulnar drift** [UL-nar drift] alteration in the position of the metacarpophalangeal joints where the fingers curve toward the ulnar bone of the forearm; results from rheumatoid arthritis

**ultra-** [ul-trah] *prefix*; extreme, beyond, or disproportionate

**ultrasonogram** [ul-trah-SON-oh-gram] use of sound waves to assess the body structures and create computerized images for study

**ultrasound** [UL-trah-sownd] noninvasive procedure that generates images via computer analysis to assess blood-flow velocity, direction, and occlusions; uses a transducer, which is placed over the blood vessel, and a computer, which analyzes the echoes for aberrations

**umbilical cord** [um-BIL-ih-kul kord] a vascular structure attaching the fetus to the placenta in utero

**umbilicate** [um-BIL-ih-KAYT] having the appearance of being pitted or indented; shaped like an umbilicus; used to describe some skin conditions

**umbilicus** [um-bih-LIE-kus] depressed point on the surface of the abdomen where the umbilical cord was formerly attached

**uni-** [yoo-nee] *prefix*; one, singular

**unigravida** [yoo-nee-GRAV-ih-da] a woman who is pregnant for the first time

**unilateral** [yoo-nih-LAT-er-ahl] confined to one side

**universal precautions** [yoo-nih-VER-sal pre-KAW-shuns] standard measures to prevent exposure to blood-borne pathogens

**Unna's boot** [YOO-naz boot] a dressing applied to stasis ulcers of the lower leg using layers of gauze and a mixture of zinc oxide in a glycogelatin base

**unremarkable** [un-re-MARK-uh-bul] no significance or information worth noting, all normal findings

**upper gastrointestinal series (UGI)** [UP-err gas-troh-en-TES-tih-nal SEER-eez] study of the esophagus, stomach, and sometimes small bowel after swallowing barium sulfate solution

**uraniscoplasty** [yoo-rayn-is-KOH-plas-tee] surgical repair of a cleft palate

**uraniscus** [yoo-ran-IS-kus] palate or roof of the mouth

**uranoplegia** [yoo-rah-noh-PLEE-jee-ah] paralysis of the soft palate of the mouth

**uremia** [yoo-REE-mee-ah] excessive urea and nitrogenous wastes in the blood

**uremic frost** [yoo-REE-mik frawst] skin appears powdery as a result of severe uremia due to dermal deposits of urea and uric acid salt

**ureter** [YOO-reh-tur] one of two small tubes that drain urine from the kidneys to the bladder

**ureteritis** [yoo-ree-ter-EYE-tis] inflammation of the ureter

**ureterocystostomy** [yoo-ree-tur-oh-SIS-TOS-tuh-mee] surgical connection made between the ureter and the bladder

**urethra** [yoo-REE-thra] the short vessel used for the purpose of eliminating or passing urine

**urethritis** [yoo-ree-THRIGH-tis] inflammation of the urethra caused by infection or mechanical irritation associated with a stone

**urethroplasty** [yoo-REE-throh-PLAS-tee] surgical procedure that involves plastic surgery to reposition the urethra; used to correct congenital hypospadias or epispadias

**-uria** [yoo-ree-ah] *suffix*; pertaining to urine or urination

**uric acid** [YOO-rik AS-id] an end product of protein metabolism that is present in measurable quantities and ultimately excreted in urine

**uricosuria** [yoo-ri-koh-SOO-ree-ah] presence of abnormal amounts of uric acid in the urine

**urinalysis** [yoo-ri-NAL-ih-sis] examination of the urine

**urinary sand** [YOOR-ih-nair-ee sand] passage of multiple minute, non-obstructing calculous particles in the urine following nephrolithiasis

**urinary tract** [YOOR-ih-nair-ee trakt] structures leading from the urinary pelvis of the kidney, ureters, and bladder to the urethra

**urine amylase test** [YOOR-un AM-il-ace] test measuring pancreatic urine levels of amylase

**urine ketosteroid tests** [YOOR-un kee-toh-STEER-oid tests] analyses of urine to detect androgen metabolites

**urine turbidity** [YOOR-in tur-BID-ih-tee] refers to the clarity of liquid excreted by the kidney

**urinophil** [YOO-rih-noh-fil] organisms such as bacteria that thrive in the urinary bladder or urine

**urochrome** [YOOR-oh-krome] yellow pigment found in urine

**urodynia** [yoo-roh-DIN-ee-ah] painful urination; often associated with urinary tract infection

**urologist** [yoo-RAWL-oh-ist] a licensed physician who specializes in the treatment of disorders of the urinary tract

**urticaria** [ur-tih-KAR-ee-ah] hives marked by redness and swelling wheals

**-us** [us] *suffix*; structure or thing

**uterine cavity** [YOO-ter-in KAV-ih-tee] hollow space within the uterus

**uterine fibroids** [YOO-ter-in FYE-broidz] benign muscle tumor of the uterus; also known as fibroids, aromas, myomas, leiomyoma, or fibromyomas

**uterine inertia** [YOO-ter-in in-ER-shah] lack of effective contractions during labor

**uterine lining** [YOO-ter-in LYN-ing] endometrial tissue

**uterine prolapse** [YOO-ter-in PRO-laps] protrusion or displacement of the uterus through the vaginal canal; assigned stages one to three depending on how far into the vaginal canal the uterus has fallen

**uterovesical** [YOO-ter-oh-VES-ik-ahl] pertaining to the uterus and bladder

**uterus** [YOO-ter-us] hollow muscular organ of the female reproductive tract where a fertilized ovum implants and develops into a fetus

**uveal tract** [YOO-vee-ahl TRAKT] collective term for the ciliary body of the eye; also known as the uvea

**uvula** [YOO-voo-lah] the fleshy hanging part of the soft palate that activates the gag reflex when stimulated

**uvulopalatopharyngoplasty** [YOO-voo-lo-PAL-ah-toh-FAIR-in-go-plas-tee] plastic surgical procedure to remove excess soft palate, uvula, and other structures of the throat to resolve sleep apnea and intractable snoring

**vaccination** [VAK-sih-NAY-shun] medical procedure that injects a vaccine into the body

**vaccine** [vak-SEEN] killed or attenuated bacterial or viral cells or cell fragments used to trigger the production of antibodies and memory B lymphocytes specific to that pathogen; routinely used to prevent diseases; also known as immunization

**vagal nerve stimulation** [VAY-gal nerv stim-yoo-LAY-shun] treatment of intractable seizure disorder where electrical impulses are delivered in 30-second segments every five minutes by a device implanted in the anterior wall

**vagina** [vah-JYN-ah] the musculomembranous tube that connects the cervix uteri and the vulva

**vaginomycosis** [VAJ-in-oh-migh-KOH-sis] fungal infection of the vagina

**vagolysis** [vay-go-LY-sis] surgical destruction of the vagus (X) nerve interrupting the impulses transmitted to the stomach and intestines

**valgus** [VAL-gus] structural deformation of being bent or turned outward; most often used to describe extremities

**Valsalva maneuver** [val-SAHL-vuh ma-NEW-vur] forced expiratory effort

**valvuloplasty** [VALV-yoo-loh-PLAS-tee] dilation of a heart valve to relieve stenosis by balloon dilatation during cardiac catheterization or surgery

**vanillylmandelic acid** [VAN-ih-lil-man-DEL-ik AS-id] the urinary metabolite that is elevated in patients with pheochromocytoma

**vaporizer** [VAY-por-iz-er] a device for changing liquid medications to a gaseous state for the purpose of inhalation

**varicocelectomy** [VAR-ih-koh-see-LEK-toh-mee] surgical excision of the scrotal sac and dilated veins

**varicose** [VAR-ih-kose] veins that are knotted or swollen; they often occur in the lower legs and esophagus due to defective vein valves; plural is varix

**varus** [VAR-us] condition in which the hind foot turns inward; usually associated with clubfoot

**vasa recta** [VAH-sa REK-tah] capillary network of a nephron in the kidney

**vasa vasorum** [VAH-sa vah-SOH-rum] minute blood vessels in the walls of larger arteries and veins

**vascular aneurysm** [VAS-kew-lur AN-yoo-riz-um] sac-shaped outward bulge on an artery

**vascular murmur** [VAS-kew-lur MUR-mur] turbulent blood flow due to incomplete closure of heart

**vascular stasis** [VAS-kyoo-lar STA-sis] pooling of blood in the periphery

**vascular stent** [VAS-kyoo-lar stent] intravascular insertion of a tubular meshwork to keep an artery open

**vascularization]** [VAS-kyoo-lar-eye-ZAY-shun] development of new blood vessels in tissue such as the myocardium

**vasectomy** [vas-EK-toh-mee] surgical procedure involving bilateral surgical removal of part of the vas deferens for the purpose of sterilization

**vasoconstriction** [vays-oh-kon-STRIK-shun] decrease in the diameter of a blood vessel

**vasodilators** [vayz-oh-dye-LAY-tors] drugs that widen blood vessels, decreasing blood pressure

**vastus intermedius muscle** [VAS-tus in-tur-MEE-dee-us MUS-sel] muscle of the anterior thigh covering the femoral shaft, situated between the vastus lateralis and vastus medialis; it functions to extends the lower leg

**vastus lateralis muscle** [VAS-tus lat-ur-AL-is MUS-sel] largest muscle of the anterior lateral aspect of the femoral shaft that extends the lower leg; often used for injection site

**vastus medialis muscle** [VAS-tus mee-dee-AL-is MUS-sel] muscle of the anterior thigh situated on the interior aspect of the femoral shaft that extends the lower leg

**vein sclerosing** [vayn skle-ROWS-ing] injection of a hypertonic solution, causing the vein to harden and eventually atrophy

**vein stripping** [vayn STRIP-ing] surgical removal of a vein after ligation of varicose veins

**veins** [VAYNZ] vessels carrying blood toward the heart

**venipuncture** [VEN-ih-punk-chur] piercing a venous blood vessel for the purpose of obtaining a blood sample

**venography** [vee-NOG-rah-fee] x-ray examination of the veins after injection of dye that absorbs the x-rays

**venostasis** [vee-noh-STAY-sis] method of reducing the amount of blood returning to the heart by compression of veins in the periphery

**ventilator** [VEN-tih-lay-tor] any of several devices used in respiratory therapy to provide assisted respiration and intensive positive-pressure breathing

**ventral** [VEN-tral] front

**-ventral** [ven-tral] *suffix*; pertaining to the stomach or abdominal area

**ventral phimosis** [VEN-tral figh-MOH-sis] stenosis of the penis prepuce

**ventral ramus** [VEN-tral RAY-mus] a branch of the spinal nerve that supplies nervous impulses to the lateral portions of the body wall, ribs, and perineum

**ventral root** [VEN-tral root] the nerve tract that connects the spinal cord to motor neurons and transmits impulses to muscles, producing movement

**ventricle** [VEN-trih-kel] a space or chamber in an organ; for example, the lower chambers of the heart

**ventricular assist device** [ven-TRIK-yoo-lar ah-SIST dee-VYS] a mechanical device that supports or replaces the function of the right or left ventricle of the heart in clients with severely diseased or nonfunctioning heart muscle

**ventricular fibrillation** [ven-TRIK-yoo-lar fib-ril-LAY-shun] rapid but ineffective movements of the ventricles of the heart that replace coordinated contractions, resulting in grossly diminished cardiac output

**ventricular hypertrophy** [ven-TRIK-yoo-lar hy-PER-troh-fee] pathological enlargement of the ventricles of the heart; often associated with valve disease, heart failure, or hypertension

**ventricular septal defect** [ven-TRIK-yoo-lur SEP-tul DEE-fekt] an abnormal opening between the ventricles, allowing blood to shunt back and forth

**ventriculoperitoneal shunt** [ven-TRIK-yoo-loh-per-it-oh-NEE-al shunt] surgical placement of tubing in the cerebral ventricle, tube has one-way valves to drain excess cerebrospinal fluid from the brain to treat hydrocephalus

**venules** [VAYN-yoolz] smallest branches of veins

**vermiform appendix** [VER-mih-form ah-PEN-diks] a wormlike intestinal diverticulum located at the end of the cecum and terminating in a blind extremity

**vermilion border** [ver-MIL-yon BOR-dur] the pink-red border around the lips

**vermis** [VUR-mis] lobe of the cerebellum between the two hemispheres

**verruca vulgaris** [ver-ROO-kuh vul-GAIR-us] common wart; caused by viral infection of the skin

**vertebrae** [VER-teh-bree] individual bones of the spinal column

**vertebral column** [VER-teh-bral KOL-um] collective name for the cervical, thoracic, lumbar and sacral bones of the dorsal spine

**vertical transmission** [VER-tih-cal trans-MIH-shun] passage of disease from the mother to the fetus during the period of pregnancy

**vertigo** [VER-tih-goh] dizziness while not moving, and ringing in the ears in quiet environments

**vesical** [VES-ih-kal] pertaining to the urinary bladder

**vesicles** [VES-ih-kuls] blisters that leak fluid

**vesicoureteral reflux** [VEZ-ih-koh-yoo-REE-ter-al REE-fluks] retrograde flow of urine from the bladder into the ureter

**vesicovaginal fistula** [ves-ih-koh-VA-jin-ahl FIS-tyoo-lah] an abnormal opening between the bladder and vagina

**vestibule** [VES-tih-byool] chamber of the inner ear

**vibices** [VYE-bi-seez] bruising in a linear pattern on the skin

**villi** [VILL-eye] projections from the surface of the gastric mucosa

**viral hepatitis** [VYE-ral hep-ah-TYE-tis] inflammation of the liver due to a viral infection

**viral load** [VYE-ral lohd] plasma measurement of viral RNA, usually done in serial fashion with human immunodeficiency disorder

**virilism** [VIR-il-izm] development of male secondary sex characteristics in a female

**virulent** [VIR-yoo-lens] highly toxic or intense disease-producing quality of a pathogen

**viscera** [VIS-er-ah] all of the internal organs of the various body cavities

**visceral muscle** [VIS-er-al MUS-sel] smooth muscle of the internal organs

**visceral pericardium** [VIS-eh-ral perr-ih-KAHR-dee-um] layer directly on the outside of the heart muscle

**viscid** [VIS-kid] a thick and sticky substance; for example, mucus secretions

**viscosity** [vis-KAWS-ih-tee] the resistance of a substance to change in shape or flow due to molecular cohesion; most often applied to liquids

**visual cortex** [VIZH-yoo-ahl KOR-teks] areas in the right and left occipital lobes of the brain that merge images from both eyes to create a single image that is right side up and in its original horizontal direction

**vital capacity (VC)** [VYE-tal kah-PAS-ih-tee] the maximum volume of air that can be exhaled following the deepest inhalation; calculated as: tidal volume + inspiratory reserve volume + expiratory reserve volume; average value = 4,500 cc

**vital signs** [VYE-tal sighns] objective measures of key body parameters, such as temperature, breathing rate, pulse, and blood pressure

**vitiligo** [vit-ih-LYE-go] skin disease characterized by patches without pigmentation

**vitrectomy** [vih-TREK-toh-mee] removing the vitreous humor and replacing it with a synthetic substitute

**vitreous humor** [VIT-ree-us HYOO-mor] clear, gel-like substance that fills the posterior cavity of the eye

**vocal fremitus** [VOL-kal FREM-ih-tus] palpable vibration in the chest wall produced by voice sounds due to consolidates or congestion

**voiding cystourethrography** [VOY-ding SIS-toh-YOO-ree-THRAWG-rah-fee] radiographic examination of the bladder before, during, and after voiding

**voluntary muscle** [VAWL-un-tar-ee MUS-sel] skeletal muscles that contract or relax in response to conscious thought

**volvulus** [VOLV-yoo-lus] twisting of a loop of intestine around itself or around another segment of bowel, causing obstruction

**vomer** [VOH-mer] a narrow wafer of bone that forms the inferior part of the nasal septum that continues posteriorly to the cranium, where it joins the sphenoid bone

**vomicose** [VOM-ih-kose] condition of having many ulcers with purulent drainage

**vomitus** [VOHM-ih-tus] expelled food or chyme

**vulvar carcinoma** [VUL-var kar-sin-OH-mah] malignant neoplasm of the vulva, most often squamous cell type, with the greatest incidence in women ages 65–70 years

**vulvorectal** [vul-voh-REK-tal] pertaining to the vulva and rectal area

# W

**wave lithotripsy** [wayv lith-oh-TRIP-see] fragmentation of stones using ultrasound short waves so that the pulverized pieces can pass naturally

**Weber test for hearing** [WEH-ber TEST for HEER-ing] assessment of bone conduction of sound by placing a vibrating tuning fork at the midpoint of the forehead to determine if sound is heard equally in both ears

**Wernicke's aphasia** [VER-nih-keez ah-FAY-zee-uh] deficit in ability to comprehend sounds or written words due to damage to the temporal lobe by trauma or stroke

**Wernicke's encephalopathy** [VER-nih-keez en-sef-ah-LOP-ah-thee] brain damage with gross short-term memory disruption due to chronic alcoholism and thiamine deficiency

**wet gangrene** [wet GANG-green] ischemia and necrosis of tissue with bacterial infection causing cellulitis in adjacent tissues

**wheal** [WHEEL] swellings in specific skin areas

**wheezes** [WHEE-zes] audible whistling breath sound often associated with asthma or airway constriction

**white matter** [whyt MAT-ter] the tissue of the central nervous system consisting mainly of myelinated nerve fibers

**Wilms tumor** [VILMS tu-mor] a rapidly developing malignant neoplasm of the kidney of unknown etiology, seen in infants and children before age five; it may be treated with surgery, radiation, or chemotherapy

**windowing** [WIN-dow-ing] to cut a hole in a cast or other material to relieve pressure on the skin or a bony prominence

**withdrawal syndrome** [with-DRAWL SIN-drom] uncomfortable physical symptoms that occur when use of a sedative, pain drug, or illegal narcotic is stopped suddenly in a patient who is physically tolerant

**word salad** [word SAL-ad] speech that includes a jumble of seemingly unrelated words; often associated with thought disorders such as schizophrenia

# X

**xanthoma** [zan-THO-muh] fat-filled cells in subcutaneous tissue

**xeno-** [zee-noh] *prefix*; strange or odd

**xenograft** [ZEN-oh-graft] tissue graft from a distant species

**xeroderma** [zeer-oh-DUR-mah] extremely dry skin

**xeroderma pigmentosum** [zeer-oh-DUR-mah pig-men-TOH-sum] abnormal skin-thickening caused by viral infection

**xerophthalmia** [ZEER-opf-THAL-mee-ah] insufficient production of tears because of eye irritation, associated aging process, or an ectropion of the eyelid

**x-rays** [EKS-rayz] use of electromagnetic radiation to penetrate body parts and produce images used for diagnosis and treatment of a wide variety of conditions

**xyphoid process** [ZY-foyd PRAW-sess] the small tip at the inferior end of the sternum

# Y

**-y** [ee] *suffix*; condition or process

**Yankauer suction catheter** [YAWN-kur SUK-shun KATH-eh-ter] a rigid, plastic-tipped device used to aspirate secretions from the mouth and throat

**yolk sack** [yohk sak] embryonic membranous tissue that produces the first red blood cell of the embryo

# Z

**Zollinger-Ellison syndrome** [ZOL-in-jer EL-ih-sun SIN-drom] hypersecretion of gastric acid and formation of gastric ulcers; associated with nonbeta cell tumors of the pancreatic isles

**zoonosis** [zoh-oh-NO-sis] spread of disease from animals to humans

**Z-plasty** [zee-PLAS-tee] use of a Z-shaped surgical incision to reduce tension on a scar produced by normal movement of a body part

**z-track method** [ZEE-trak METH-od] a technique of administering an intramuscular injection that prevents the fluid from seeping out of the site by pulling the skin tightly to one side, administering the injection, removing the needle, then allowing the skin to slide back into the normal position

**zygomatic bones** [ZY-goh-mah-tik bohnz] facial bones that form the lateral edges of the eye sockets and cheekbones

**zygomaticus muscle** [zye-goh-MAT-ih-kus MUS-sel] the facial muscle that draws the corner of the mouth upward and outward

**zygote** [ZYE-gote] a fertilized ovum

# Resource Lists

**2**

> ## RESOURCE CATEGORY 1: ANATOMY/PHYSIOLOGY

*Figure 1:* Arterial Supply to the Heart

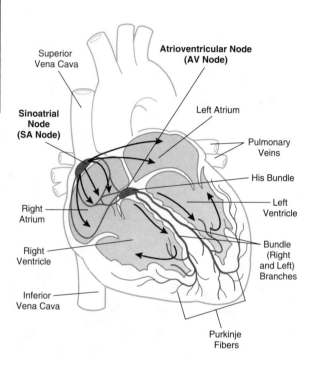

*Figure 2:* Cardiac Conduction System

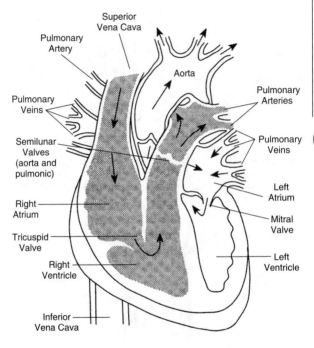

*Figure 3:* Cardiovascular System, Heart

*Figure 4:* Cardiovascular System, Major Veins

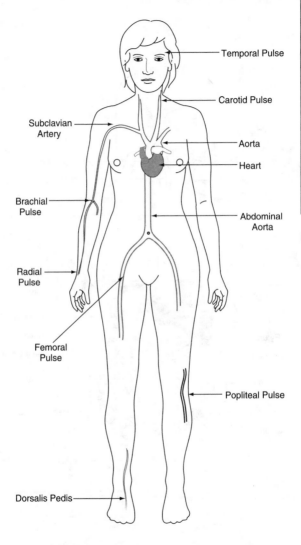

Temporal Pulse

Carotid Pulse

Subclavian Artery

Aorta

Heart

Brachial Pulse

Abdominal Aorta

Radial Pulse

Femoral Pulse

Popliteal Pulse

Dorsalis Pedis

*Figure 5:* Cardiovascular System, Pulse Points

*Figure 6:* Digestive System

*Figure 7:* Endocrine System

*Figure 8:* Excretory System

*Figure 9:* Human Fetus

*Figure 10:* Lymph Node

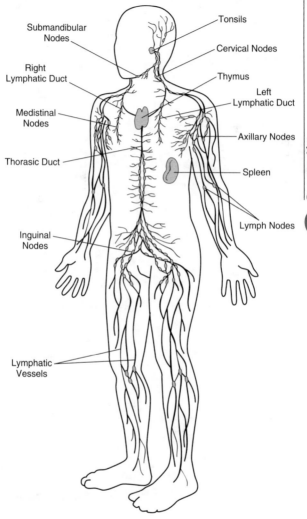

Submandibular Nodes

Right Lymphatic Duct

Medistinal Nodes

Thorasic Duct

Inguinal Nodes

Lymphatic Vessels

Tonsils

Cervical Nodes

Thymus

Left Lymphatic Duct

Axillary Nodes

Spleen

Lymph Nodes

*Figure 11:* Lymphatic System

*Figure 12:* Muscles, Anterior

*Figure 13:* Muscles, Posterior

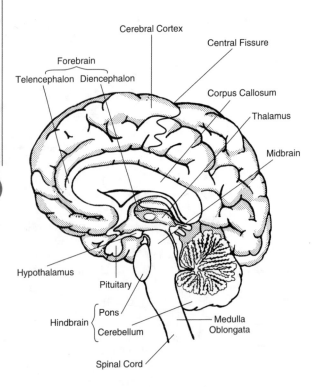

Cerebral Cortex

Central Fissure

Forebrain

Telencephalon    Diencephalon

Corpus Callosum

Thalamus

Midbrain

Hypothalamus

Pituitary

Pons

Hindbrain

Cerebellum

Medulla
Oblongata

Spinal Cord

*Figure 14:* Nervous System, Brain

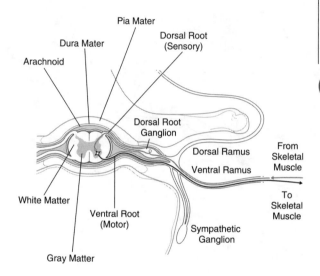

*Figure 15:* Nervous System, Cross-Section of Spinal Cord and
the Components of a Spinal Nerve

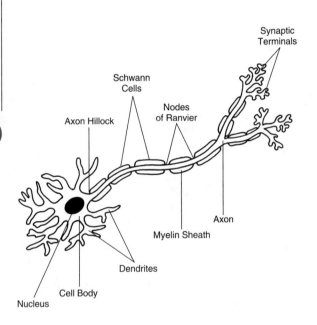

*Figure 16:* Nervous System, Neuron

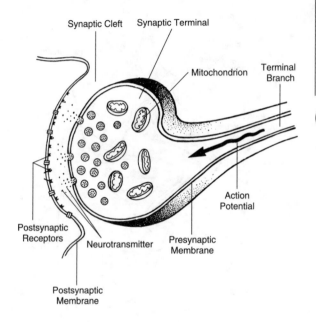

*Figure 17:* Nervous System, Synapse

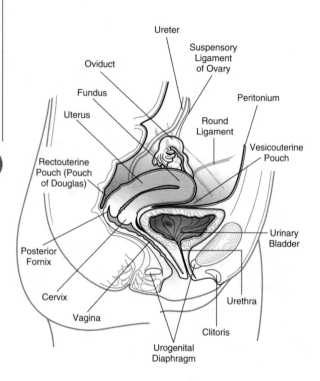

*Figure 18:* Reproductive System, Female

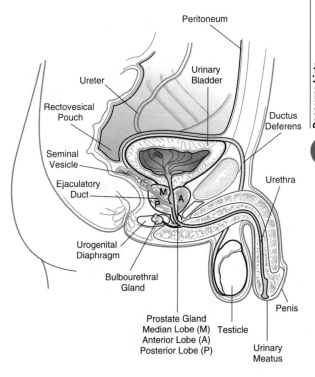

*Figure 19:* Reproductive System, Male

*Figure 20:* Respiratory System

*Figure 21:* Skeletal System, Bones

A. Transverse: Break across Entire Cross-Section of Bone

B. Incomplete: Break through Portion of Bone

C. Closed: No External Communication

D. Compound: Extends through Skin

E. Colles Fracture

F. Greenstick Fracture

G. Depressed Skull Fracture

H. Pott's Fracture

*Figure 22:* Skeletal System, Fractures

1. Lateral View
   Body
   Pedicle

2. Posterior View

3. Annulus Fibrosus
   Nucleus Pulposus

4. Intervertebral Disk
   Intervertebral Foramen
   Zygapophyseal Joint
   Spinal Nerve
   Anterior Ligament
   Posterior Longitudinal Ligament

*Figure 23:* Skeletal System, Intervertebral Foramen

*Figure 24:* Skin

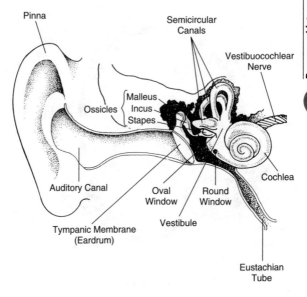

Pinna

Semicircular
Canals

Vestibuocochlear
Nerve

Ossicles

Malleus
Incus
Stapes

Auditory Canal

Oval
Window

Round
Window

Cochlea

Tympanic Membrane
(Eardrum)

Vestibule

Eustachian
Tube

*Figure 25:* Special Sense Organs, Ear

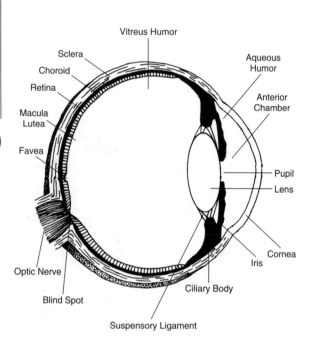

*Figure 26:* Special Sense Organs, Eye

## ➤ RESOURCE CATEGORY 2: DISEASES, DISORDERS, AND PROCEDURES

### General Pathology

#### Neurological Disorders

acetylcholine
agnosia
agraphia
Alzheimer's disease
amyotrophic lateral sclerosis
aphagia
aphasia
apraxia
Asperger's disorder
athetosis
autism
Babinski sign
Bell's palsy
cataplexy
catastrophic reaction
cerebral palsy
circumstantiality
cognition
concussion
coup-contre coup
delirium
delirium tremens
dementia
encephalitis
Erb palsy
Huntington chorea
hydrocephalus
Lewy body dementia
multi-infarct dementia
multiple sclerosis
myasthenia gravis
progressive supranuclear palsy
punch drunk syndrome
seizure
tonic-clonic movements
Wernicke syndrome

#### Cancer

adenocarcinoma
antineoplastics
astrocytoma
basal cell carcinoma
chemotherapy
Cheyne-Stokes respirations
dyscrasia
ependymoma
Ewing's sarcoma
hepatoma
inguinodynia
lymphadenopathy

lymphangioma
lymphoma
medulloblastoma
metastasize
myelogenous leukemia
neoplasm
neoplastic
nephroblastoma
osteosarcoma

palliative care
patient-controlled analgesia
polyadenoma
precancerous
radiation therapy
rhabdomyosarcoma
squamous cell carcinoma
T cells
tumor suppressor genes

## COPD

antitussives
arterial blood gases
bronchodilator
circumoral cyanosis
clubbing of fingers
cough
cyanosis
effusion
emphysema
empyema
endotoxin
endotracheal intubation
epinephrine
expectorate
expiratory reserve volume

extubation
hemoptysis
hypercapnia
hypoglycemia
incentive spirometry
intercostal retractions
mucolytic
mucopurulent
nebulizer
perfusion
pulse oximeter
sepsis
tracheobronchial suction
vaporizer
vocal fremitus

## Respiratory Diseases

acute respiratory distress
    syndrome
antihistamines
aspiration pneumonia
assist-control ventilation
asthma

atelectasis
bag-valve-mask
bronchial asthma
bronchiectasis
bronchitis
bronchodilators

bronchopneumonia
bronchospasm
chest physiotherapy
controlled mandatory
    ventilation
empyema
hyaline membrane disease
hyperresonance
mechanical ventilation
oligopnea

peak expiratory flow
pleural effusion
pleuralgia
pneumocentesis
pneumoconiosis
*Pneumocystis carinii*
pneumonia
pneumothorax
pulmonary atresio
pyothorax

## Diabetes

alkalosis
amylase
antidiabetic drugs
atonic bladder
diabetes insipidus
diabetes mellitus
diabetes mellitus, type I
diabetes mellitus, type II
diabetes neuropathy
diabetic ketoacidosis
diabetic retinopathy
fructosuria
glucagon
glucometer
glucosuria
glycohemoglobin

glycosylated hemoglobin
hyperinsulinism
hypoglycemia
hyposecretion
insulin resistance
insulin shock
ketonuria
metabolic syndrome
neurogenic bladder
oral antidiabetic
pancreas
pancreatic islets
pancreatography
polydipsia
retinopathy

## Heart Disease

aberrant conduction
angiospasm
angiostenosis
aortalgia

aortic stenosis
asynchronous pacing
atherosclerotic plaque
atrial ectopic beats

atrial fibrillation
atrial septal defect
cardiomyopathy
cardioplegia
cardioversion
carotid sinus syndrome
coarctation of the aorta
congestive heart disease
congestive heart failure
cor pulmonale
coronary bypass
digitalization
dissecting aneurysm
ejection murmur
endopericarditis
hyperlipidemia
implanted cardioverter
    defibrillator

intermittent claudication
mitral valve prolapse
myocardial infarction
myocarditis
neoplastic heart syndrome
pacing catheter
phlebothrombosis
premature atrial contractions
pulmonic stenosis
sinus tachycardia
supraventricular tachycardia
tissue plasminogen
    activator
tricuspid atresia
vascular stent
ventricular fibrillation
ventricular hypertrophy

## Parkinson's Disease

anosmia
anticholinergics
astasia
asterixis
asthenia
ataxia
bradykinesia
bradyphrasia
cerebellar gait
cogwheeling
dopamine
dyskinesia
dysphagia
dysphonia
dystonia

extrapyramidal side effects
gait apraxia
hypokinetic dysarthria
myoclonus
neuroleptic
oculogyric crisis
pallidotomy
Parkinson facies
rigidity
sialorrhea
somnolent
tardive dyskinesia
torpid
tremor

## Sexually Transmitted Diseases

acquired immunodeficiency syndrome (AIDS)
amebiasis
bacterial vaginosis
balanitis
chancroid
*Chlamydia trachomatis*
colposcope
condyloma acuminatum
cryptosporidiosis
cystitis
cytomegalovirus
giardiasis
gonorrhea
hepatitis A
hepatitis B
hepatitis C
herpes simplex
human papilloma virus
Kaposi's sarcoma
lymphogranuloma venereum
molluscum contagiosum
pelvic inflammatory disease
proctocolitis
protease inhibitor drugs
scabies
sexually transmitted disease
syphilis
viral load
vulvar carcinoma

## Stroke

anisocoria
aphagia
aphasia
asaphia
atony
atrophy
bradyglossia
cerebral angiography
cerebral edema
cerebral perfusion pressure
cerebrovascular accident
coma
contracture
decerebrate rigidity
dystonia
enteral nutrition
flaccid
Glasgow coma scale
hemianopia
hemiparesis
hemiplegia
hemorrhagic stroke
ischemic stroke
monoplegia
paralysis
paresthesia
phlebosclerosis
phrenoplegia
thrombolytic therapy
transient ischemic attack

## Procedures

### Diagnostic

air-puff tonometry
alanine aminotransferase
    test
angiogram
arthrogram
barium enema
biopsy
bone densitometry
bone marrow aspiration
cardiac catheterization
cardiac scan
colposcopy
computerized axial
    tomography
culdocentesis
digital subtraction
    angiography
dilated funduscopy
echocardiogram

electrocardiogram
electroencephalograph
endoscopic retrograde
    cholangiopancreatography
fluorescein angiography
fluoroscopy
lumbar puncture
magnetic resonance
    imaging
pulmonary function tests
pulmonary ventilation scan
radioactive iodine uptake
    test
radionuclide scan
scintigraphy
single-photon emission
    computed tomography
thyroid scan
voiding cystourethrography

### Surgical

adrenalectomy
angioplasty
appendectomy
bladder neck suspension
cardiopulmonary bypass graft
cecocolopexy
chondrectomy
colpoperineoplasty
craniotomy
cystostomy

dacryocystorhinostomy
endarterectomy
enterocolectomy
ganglionectomy
gastrectomy
hemicolectomy
hysterectomy
ileotomy
laryngectomy
laryngotracheotomy

laser-assisted in situ
keratomileusis
lymphangioplasty
myringotomy
orchidoplasty
polypectomy
prostatectomy
radical neck dissection
rhizotomy

salpingo oophorectomy
splenectomy
tendoplasty
thoracotomy
trabeculoplasty
ureterocystostomy
valvuloplasty
ventriculoperitoneal shunt

## ➤ RESOURCE CATEGORY 3:
## WORD ROOTS, PREFIXES, AND SUFFIXES

### Word Roots

*Note: These are listed in their combining form.*

abdomin/o
arthr/o
cardi/o
colon/o
crani/o
cutane/o
cyst/o
cyt/o
derm/o
enter/o
gastr/o
hemat/o
hepat/o
hyster/o
lith/o

muscul/o
my/o
neph/ro
neur/o
oophor/o
orchid/o
oste/o
phleb/o
rhin/o
therm/o
thorac/o
troph/o
tympan/o
ventr/o
vesic/o

## Prefixes

ab-
ad-
allo-
an-
apo-
auto-
brachy-
brady-
contra-
dis-
dys-
ec-
ecto-
endo-
epi-

eu-
heme-
hyper-
hypo-
infra-
intra-
iso-
macro-
neo-
oto-
pan-
per-
supra-
tachy-
xeno-

## Suffixes

-al
-ase
-asthenia
-ate
-blast
-cele
-centesis
-cephalus
-cle
-derma
-desis
-dynia
-eal
-ectasis
-ectomy

-emia
-entery
–gravida
-ic
-ism
-itis
-lith
-lysis
-ole
-oma
-phil
-plasia
-plasty
-rrhaphy
-rrhea

# Medical Abbreviations

## 3

## ➤ COMMON MEDICAL ABBREVIATIONS

**ABC**   airway, breathing, circulation
**abd.**   abdomen
**ABG**   arterial blood gas
**ABO**   system of classifying blood groups
**ac**   before meals
**ACE**   angiotensin converting enzyme
**ACS**   acute compartment syndrome
**ACTH**   adrenocorticotrophic hormone
**ADH**   antidiuretic hormone
**ADL**   activities of daily living
**ad lib**   freely, as desired
**AFP**   alpha-fetoprotein
**AIDS**   acquired immunodeficiency syndrome
**AKA**   above the knee amputation
**ALL**   acute lymphocytic leukemia
**ALS**   amyotrophic lateral sclerosis
**ALT**   alkaline phosphatase (formerly SGPT)
**AMI**   antibody-mediated immunity
**AML**   acute myelogenous leukemia
**amt.**   amount
**ANA**   antinuclear antibody
**ANS**   autonomic nervous system
**AP**   anteroposterior
**A&P**   anterior and posterior

**APC** atrial premature contraction
**aq.** water
**ARDS** adult respiratory distress syndrome
**ASD** atrial septal defect
**ASHD** atherosclerotic heart disease
**AST** aspartate aminotransferase (formerly SGOT)
**ATP** adenosine triphosphate
**AV** atrioventricular
**BCG** Bacille Calmette-Guerin
**bid** two times a day
**BKA** below the knee amputation
**BLS** basic life support
**BMR** basal metabolic rate
**BP** blood pressure
**BPH** benign prostatic hypertrophy
**bpm** beats per minute
**BPR** bathroom privileges
**BSA** body surface area
**BUN** blood, urea, nitrogen
**C** centigrade, Celsius
**c̄** with
**Ca** calcium
**CA** cancer
**CABG** coronary artery bypass graft
**CAD** coronary artery disease
**CAPD** continuous ambulatory peritoneal dialysis
**caps** capsules
**CBC** complete blood count
**CC** chief complaint
**CCU** coronary care unit, critical care unit
**CDC** Centers for Disease Control and Prevention
**CHF** congestive heart failure
**CK** creatine kinase
**Cl** chloride
**CLL** chronic lymphocytic leukemia
**cm** centimeter
**CMV** cytomegalovirus infection

**CNS** central nervous system
**CO** carbon monoxide, cardiac output
**CO$_2$** carbon dioxide
**comp** compound
**cont** continuous
**COPD** chronic obstructive pulmonary disease
**CP** cerebral palsy
**CPAP** continuous positive airway pressure
**CPK** creatine phosphokinase
**CPR** cardiopulmonary resuscitation
**CRP** C-reactive protein
**C&S** culture and sensitivity
**CSF** cerebrospinal fluid
**CT** computerized tomography
**CTD** connective tissue disease
**CTS** carpal tunnel syndrome
**cu** cubic
**CVA** cerebrovascular accident or costovertebral angle
**CVC** central venous catheter
**CVP** central venous pressure
**DC** discontinue
**D&C** dilation and curettage
**DIC** disseminated intravascular coagulation
**DIFF** differential blood count
**dil.** dilute
**DJD** degenerative joint disease
**DKA** diabetic ketoacidosis
**dl** deciliter (100 ml)
**DM** diabetes mellitus
**DNA** deoxyribonucleic acid
**DNR** do not resuscitate
**DO** doctor of osteopathy
**DOE** dyspnea on exertion
**DPT** vaccine for diphtheria, pertussis, tetanus
**Dr.** doctor
**DVT** deep vein thrombosis
**D/W** dextrose in water

**Dx**   diagnosis

**ECF**   extracellular fluid

**ECG or EKG**   electrocardiogram

**ECT**   electroconvulsive therapy

**ED**   emergency department

**EEG**   electroencephalogram

**EMD**   electromechanical dissociation

**EMG**   electromyography

**ENT**   ear, nose, and throat

**ESR**   erythrocyte sedimentation rate

**ESRD**   end stage renal disease

**ET**   endotracheal tube

**F**   Fahrenheit

**FBD**   fibrocystic breast disease

**FBS**   fasting blood sugar

**FDA**   Food and Drug Administration

**FFP**   fresh frozen plasma

**fl**   fluid

**4 x 4**   piece of gauze 4" by 4" used for dressings

**FSH**   follicle-stimulating hormone

**ft.**   foot, feet (unit of measure)

**FUO**   fever of undetermined origin

**g, gm**   gram

**GB**   gallbladder

**GFR**   glomerular filtration rate

**GH**   growth hormone

**GI**   gastrointestinal

**gr**   grain

**GSC**   Glasgow coma scale

**gtts**   drops

**GU**   genitourinary

**GYN**   gynecological

**h or hrs**   hour or hours

**(H)**   hypodermically

**Hb or Hgb**   hemoglobin

**HCG**   human chorionic gonadotropin

**HCO$_3$−**   bicarbonate

**Hct** hematocrit
**HD** hemodialysis
**HDL** high-density lipoproteins
**Hg** mercury
**Hgb** hemoglobin
**HGH** human growth hormone
**HHNC** hyperglycemia hyperosmolar nonketotic coma
**HIV** human immunodeficiency virus
**HLA** human leukocyte antigen
**HR** heart rate
**hr** hour
**HSV** herpes simplex virus
**HTN** hypertension
**H₂O** water
**Hx** history
**Hz** hertz (cycles/second)
**IAPB** intra-aortic balloon pump
**IBBP** intermittent positive pressure breathing
**IBS** irritable bowel syndrome
**ICF** intracellular fluid
**ICP** increased intracranial pressure
**ICS** intercostal space
**ICU** intensive care unit
**IDDM** insulin dependent diabetes mellitus
**IgA** immunoglobulin A
**IM** intramuscular
**I&O** intake and output
**IOP** increased intraocular pressure
**IPG** impedance plethysmogram
**IPPB** intermittent positive-pressure breathing
**IUD** intrauterine device
**IV** intravenous
**IVC** intraventricular catheter
**IVP** intravenous pyelogram
**JRA** juvenile rheumatoid arthritis
**K⁺** potassium
**kcal** kilocalorie (food calorie)

**kg**   kilogram
**KO, KVO**   keep vein open
**KS**   Kaposi's sarcoma
**KUB**   kidneys, ureters, bladder
**L, l**   liter
**lab**   laboratory
**lb.**   pound
**LBBB**   left bundle branch block
**LDH**   lactate dehydrogenase
**LDL**   low-density lipoproteins
**LE**   lupus erythematosus
**LH**   luteinizing hormone
**liq**   liquid
**LLQ**   left lower quadrant
**LOC**   level of consciousness
**LP**   lumbar puncture
**LPN, LVN**   licensed practical or vocational nurse
**Lt, lt**   left
**LTC**   long term care
**LUQ**   left upper quadrant
**LV**   left ventricle
**m**   minum, meter, micron
**MAO**   monoamine oxidase inhibitors
**MAST**   military antishock trousers
**mcg**   microgram
**MCH**   mean corpuscular hemoglobin
**MCV**   mean corpuscular volume
**MD**   muscular dystrophy, medical doctor
**MDI**   metered dose inhaler
**mEq**   milliequivalent
**mg**   milligram
**Mg**   magnesium
**MG**   myasthenia gravis
**MI**   myocardial infarction
**ml**   milliliter
**mm**   millimeter
**MMR**   vaccine for measles, mumps, rubella

**MRI**   magnetic resonance imaging
**MS**   multiple sclerosis
**N**   nitrogen, normal (strength of solution)
**NIDDM**   non-insulin dependent diabetes mellitus
**Na⁺**   sodium
$Na^+$   sodium
**NaCl**   sodium chloride
**NANDA**   North American Nursing Diagnosis Association
**NG**   nasogastric
**NGT**   nasogastric tube
**NLN**   National League for Nursing
**noc**   at night
**NPO**   nothing by mouth
**NS**   normal saline
**NSAIDS**   nonsteroidal anti-inflammatory drugs
**NSNA**   National Student Nurses' Association
**NST**   non-stress test
**O₂**   oxygen
**OB-GYN**   obstetrics and gynecology
**OCT**   oxytocin challenge test
**OOB**   out of bed
**OPC**   outpatient clinic
**OR**   operating room
$\overline{os}$   by mouth
**OSHA**   Occupational Safety and Health Administration
**OTC**   over the counter (drug that can be obtained without a prescription)
**oz.**   ounce
$\overline{p}$   with
**P**   pulse, pressure, phosphorus
**PA Chest**   posterior-anterior chest x-ray
**PAC**   premature atrial complexes
**PaCO₂**   partial pressure of carbon dioxide in arterial blood
**PaO₂**   partial pressure of oxygen in arterial blood
**PAD**   peripheral artery disease
**Pap**   Papanicolaou smear
**pc**   after meals
**PCA**   patient controlled analgesia

**PCO$_2$**  partial pressure of carbon dioxide
**PCP**  Pneumocystis carinii pneumonia
**PD**  peritoneal dialysis
**PE**  pulmonary embolism
**PEEP**  positive end-expiratory pressure
**PERRLA**  pupils equal, round, react to light and accommo-
      dation
**PET**  postural emission tomography
**PFT**  pulmonary function tests
**pH**  hydrogen ion concentration
**PID**  pelvic inflammatory disease
**PKD**  polycystic disease
**PKU**  phenylketonuria
**PMS**  premenstrual syndrome
**PND**  paroxysmal nocturnal dyspnea
**PO, po**  by mouth
**PO$_2$**  partial pressure of oxygen
**PPD**  positive purified protein derivative (of tuberculin)
**PPN**  partial parenteral nutrition
**PRN, prn**  as needed, whenever necessary
**pro time**  prothrombin time
**PSA**  prostate-specific antigen
**psi**  pounds per square inch
**PSP**  phenol-sulfonphthalein
**PT**  physical therapy, prothrombin time
**PTCA**  percutaneous transluminal coronary angioplasty
**PTH**  parathyroid hormone
**PTT**  partial thromboplastin time
**PUD**  peptic ulcer disease
**PVC**  premature ventricular contraction
**q**  every
**QA**  quality assurance
**qh**  every hour
**q 2 h**  every two hours
**q 4 h**  every four hours
**qid**  four times a day
**qs**  quantity sufficient

**R** rectal temperature, respirations, roentgen
**RA** rheumatoid arthritis
**RAI** radioactive iodine
**RAIU** radioactive iodine uptake
**RAS** reticular activating system
**RBBB** right bundle branch block
**RBC** red blood cell or count
**RCA** right coronary artery
**RDA** recommended dietary allowance
**resp** respirations
**RF** rheumatic fever, rheumatoid factor
**Rh** antigen on blood cell indicated by + or –
**RIND** reversible ischemic neurologic deficit
**RLQ** right lower quadrant
**RN** registered nurse
**RNA** ribonucleic acid
**R/O, r/o** rule out, to exclude
**ROM** range of motion (of joint)
**Rt, rt** right
**RUQ** right upper quadrant
**Rx** prescription
**s̄** without
**S. or Sig.** (Signa) to write on label
**SA** sinoatrial node
**SaO₂** systemic arterial oxygen saturation (%)
**sat sol** saturated solution
**SBE** subacute bacterial endocarditis
**SDA** same day admission
**SDS** same day surgery
**sed rate** sedimentation rate
**SGOT** serum glutamic-oxaloacetic transaminase (see AST)
**SGPT** serum glutamic-pyruvic transaminase (see ALT)
**SI** International System of Units
**SIADH** syndrome of inappropriate antidiuretic hormone
**SIDS** sudden infant death syndrome
**SL** sublingual
**SLE** systemic lupus erythematosus

**SOB**  short of breath
**sol**  solution
**SMBG**  self-monitoring blood glucose
**SMR**  submucous resection
**sp gr**  specific gravity
**spec.**  specimen
$\overline{ss}$  one half
**SS**  soap suds
**SSKI**  saturated solution of potassium iodide
**stat**  immediately
**STD**  sexually transmitted disease
**subcut**  subcutaneous
**sx**  symptoms
**Syr.**  syrup
**T**  temperature, thoracic to be followed by the number
    designating specific thoracic vertebra
**T&A**  tonsillectomy and adenoidectomy
**tabs**  tablets
**TB**  tuberculosis
**T&C**  type and crossmatch
**TED**  antiembolitic stockings
**temp**  temperature
**TENS**  transcutaneous electrical nerve stimulation
**TIA**  transient ischemic attack
**TIBC**  total iron binding capacity
**tid**  three times a day
**tinct,** or **tr.**  tincture
**TMJ**  temporomandibular joint
**t-pa, TPA**  tissue plasminogen activator
**TPN**  total parenteral nutrition
**TPR**  temperature, pulse, respiration
**TQM**  total quality management
**TSE**  testicular self-examination
**TSH**  thyroid-stimulating hormone
**tsp**  teaspoon
**TSS**  toxic shock syndrome
**TURP**  transuretheral prostatectomy

**UA** urinalysis
**ung** ointment
**URI** upper respiratory tract infection
**UTI** urinary tract infection
**VAD** venous access device
**VDRL** Veneral Disease Research laboratory (test for syphilis)
**VF, Vfib** ventricular fibrillation
**VPC** ventricular premature complexes
**VS, vs** vital signs
**VSD** ventricular septal defect
**VT** ventricular tachycardia
**WBC** white blood cell or count
**WHO** World Health Organization
**wt** weight

Medical Abbreviations